2.
SUPER
FOODS

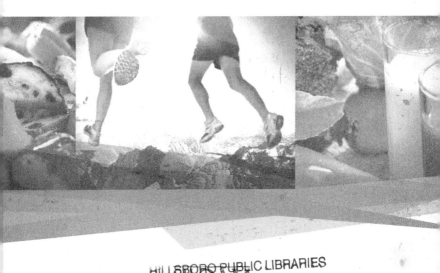

Most CHARISMA HOUSE BOOK GROUP products are available at special quantity discounts for bulk purchase for sales promotions, premiums, fund-raising, and educational needs. For details, write Charisma House Book Group, 600 Rinehart Road, Lake Mary, Florida 32746, or telephone (407) 333-0600.

21 SUPERFOODS edited by Siloam
Published by Siloam
Charisma Media/Charisma House Book Group
600 Rinehart Road
Lake Mary, Florida 32746
www.charismahouse.com

Cover design by Lisa Rae Cox
Design Director: Bill Johnson

For more information on books published by Siloam, visit www. charismahouse.com.   *5574 0616 08/14*
Library of Congress Control Number: 2014936481
International Standard Book Number: 978-1-62136-615-7
E-book ISBN: 978-1-62136-616-4

While every effort has been made to provide accurate telephone numbers and Internet addresses at the time of publication, neither the publisher nor the author assumes any responsibility for errors or for changes that occur after publication.

First edition

14 15 16 17 18 — 987654321
Printed in the United States of America

CONTENTS

Chapter 1

TERRIFIC TOMATOES

EATING CAN BE therapeutic and enjoyable if you eat the right things. And while few people likely categorize the humble tomato as a "superstar," this delicious, versatile vegetable is a healthy superfood. Whether used in salads, as the base of a hearty soup, or as a healthy topping on a vegetable pizza, tomatoes add taste and nutrition to your food without adding many calories. Even better, they are a prime cancer fighter and contain many other benefits.

Tomatoes are the best dietary source of lycopene, a primary source of bioavailable carotenoid, which gives tomatoes their bright red color. Since lycopene contains powerful antioxidants, they can counteract the effects of systematic inflammation and scavenge free radicals, which can damage cells and genes. The lycopene in tomatoes also has phytochemicals in their natural state, which are cancer inhibitors. Thus tomatoes are rich in the stuff that may prevent cancer from developing in the first place.

However, unlike many other vegetables (or fruits, if you want to be absolutely correct about it), tomatoes are not best eaten in their raw form. Tomato paste is richest in lycopene, while spaghetti sauces, ketchup, and tomato sauce have roughly half as much as the paste they are made from. From there tomato soup, canned tomatoes, and tomato juice all have about a third of the lycopene in tomato paste. Raw tomatoes have a little more than 10 percent the lycopene of tomato paste.

Tomato sauce (not ketchup) is one of the main ingredients of the healthy Mediterranean diet. It is associated with an even greater reduction in prostate cancer risk, especially for the more aggressive and life-threatening extraprostatic cancers. Harvard Medical School researchers reported in the *Journal of the National Cancer Institute* that lycopene intake was associated with reduced risk of prostate cancer.[1]

There are a number of studies that have linked lycopene with a reduced risk of prostate cancer, though these results have not been universally proven in all research done on this relationship. However, the benefits of lycopene-rich diets seem most beneficial in men most at risk for prostate cancer (those ages sixty-five and older). It seems lycopene corrects something the aging process weakens.

Research continues on the exact reasons that tomatoes aid in the fight against prostate cancer, but the correlation is strong enough—and there are enough other health benefits from sauces made from tomatoes—that adding tomato products to your diet is a smart move.

LYCOPENE'S POWERFUL IMPACT

There are other epidemiological studies showing that the regular intake of tomatoes and tomato products is associated with a lower risk of several cancers. One case-control study of an elderly population linked the consistent intake of tomato lycopene to protective effects against digestive tract cancers and a 50 percent reduction in death from cancer.[2]

Dr. Edward Giovannucci reviewed seventy-two epidemiological studies.[3] These included ecological, case-control, dietary, and blood specimen-based investigations. All the studies examined the effect of tomato lycopene on cancer. In the majority the researchers found an inverse association between tomato intake and the risk of several types of cancer. In other words, the more tomatoes a person ate, the lower his risk of getting cancer.

In thirty-five of these studies the inverse associations were statistically significant. The evidence for benefit was strongest for cancers of the prostate, lungs, and stomach. Data also suggested benefit for cancers of the pancreas, colon, rectum, esophagus, oral cavity, breast, and cervix. What's more, none of these studies showed adverse effects from high tomato intake.

Prostate cancer is the most common cancer and second leading cause of cancer mortality in men in the United States. Studies have suggested a potential benefit of tomato lycopene against the risk of prostate cancer, particularly in its more lethal forms. An 83 percent reduction of prostate cancer risk was observed in individuals with the highest plasma concentration of lycopene, compared to individuals with the lowest concentrations.[4] Eating something with tomato sauce in it as little as twice a week is thought to lower the risk of prostate cancer by around 25 percent.[5]

Recipe: Veggie Slimming Soup

2 Tbsp. olive oil

1 large onion, chopped

1 green or red bell pepper, chopped

4 garlic cloves, minced

1/2 tsp. ground cumin

1/2 small head cabbage, sliced

2 large carrots, sliced

1 zucchini, chopped

1 yellow squash, chopped

1 can (14 1/2 oz.) low-sodium stewed tomatoes

1 bottle (46 oz.) vegetable juice

1/2 tsp. ground black pepper

1/4 tsp. crushed red pepper flakes

Warm oil in a large saucepan over medium heat. Add onion and bell pepper. Cook five minutes or until tender. Add garlic and cumin. Cook one minute. Add cabbage, carrots, zucchini, squash, tomatoes (with juice), vegetable juice, black pepper, and red pepper flakes. Heat to boiling. Reduce heat to low, cover, and simmer one hour.

Lycopene Sources

Tomato sauce—including ketchup, tomato juice, and pizza sauce—is the richest source of lycopene in the American diet, accounting for greater than 80 percent of the total lycopene intake of Americans. Processed tomatoes (canned tomatoes, tomato sauce, ketchup) contain more lycopene than unprocessed tomatoes because cooking breaks down cell walls, releasing and concentrating carotenoids.

Not only has lycopene benefited Americans, habitual intake of tomato products has also been associated with the lowered risk of cancer of the digestive tract among Italians. One six-year study by Harvard Medical School and Harvard School of Public Health examined the diets of more than forty-seven thousand men. Of forty-six fruits and vegetables researchers evaluated, only the tomato products with lycopene showed a measurable relationship to a lowered risk of prostate cancer.[6] As consumption of tomato products increased, levels of lycopene in the blood increased, and the risk of prostate cancer decreased. The study showed that heat processing of tomato products increased lycopene's bioavailability, meaning that it was more easily absorbed by the body.

OTHER BENEFITS

There are other reasons to add tomatoes to your daily menu, including one not ordinarily associated with them: citrus. While citrus fruits are famous for their vitamin C—a valuable antioxidant linked to all kinds of wonderful benefits—these fruits are also among the best sources available of flavones, as well as fiber, folic acid, and potassium. And they contain limonoids, which have been shown to have powerful anti-cancer characteristics. Since these are not found in any other fruit except citrus, this gives them a unique cancer-fighting potential.

Mention "citrus," and most people think primarily of oranges, lemons, limes, and grapefruit. However, such foods as tomatoes, pineapples, kumquats, mandarin oranges, and tangerines are also high in vitamin C. Studies from around the world have repeatedly linked the consumption of citrus fruits (not juices) with a decreased risk of developing different cancers, especially those of the digestive tract: esophageal, mouth, larynx, pharynx, and stomach. Results varied, but most showed a decrease of 40 to 50 percent.[7]

Juicing Tip

Combining the juice from several tomatoes with the juice from a few slices of green bell peppers makes a great refreshing low-sodium alternative to commercial tomato juice drinks.

Tomatoes are heart healthy too, along with such superfoods as black beans, kidney beans, citrus fruits, oatmeal, green tea, and flaxseed. You will read about the healthiest in chapter 3: nuts, which in general are a beneficial part of a healthy diet. Walnuts, in particular, contain almost twice the antioxidants as other nuts.

Finally, tomatoes are a source of such minerals as potassium and silicon.

Potassium helps to lower blood pressure and keep your body's sodium at acceptable levels. That is why eating foods high in potassium, such as fresh fruits and vegetables, can help protect against high blood pressure. Tomatoes should be high on your list of high-potassium foods when you shop, along with foods such as beans (especially lima beans and soybeans), prunes, avocados, bananas, peaches, and cantaloupes.

Silicon increases the thickness and strength of skin, smooths out wrinkles, and gives hair and nails a healthier appearance. Plus, it plays a vital role in the formation of connective tissue. Consequently, it helps to maintain the elastic quality of the skin, tendons, and, generally, cell walls. You can increase your intake of silicon by consuming silicon-rich foods, such as tomatoes, cucumbers, and bell peppers (eat all three with the skin and choose organic), radishes, romaine lettuce, marjoram, and nopal cactus (prickly pear cactus).

Chapter 2

GREAT GRAPES

L IKE TOMATOES, GRAPES contain a secret healing power. They also offer a tasty way to consume enough of the fruits and vegetables that should be a part of your diet. Grapes are known for their pharmacological properties; grapes and the wines they produce contain concentrations of a class of phytochemicals called polyphenols. Although their ability to protect from cancer is well documented, at the molecular level the ways in which they do so are still unclear. However, it has been shown that grapes and grape extracts can be used as a chemopreventive agent against carcinogenesis, because:

+ They inhibit oxidative stress and show a potent anti-radical effect.

+ They suppress cell proliferation and strongly inhibit tumor growth.

+ They inhibit angiogenesis and strongly inhibit vascular endothelial growth factor, which inhibits the development of tumors and blood vessels.

+ They tend to promote apoptosis (programmed cell death) in cancer cells.

Not only do grapes have blood sugar benefits, several of their phytonutrients may play a role in extending a person's lifespan by providing maximum nutrition for fewer calories. They also abound with antioxidants, which in foods can often be identified by their bright colors—one reason to select an array of colorful grapes and other produce. The antioxidants that are found naturally in many foods, including grapes and other fruits and vegetables, nuts, grains, and some meats, include: beta-carotene, lutein, lycopene, selenium, vitamins A, C, and E.[1]

Other beneficial aspects:

* Black grapes and red grapes are among common food sources of quercetin, a plant-derived flavonoid that supports the immune system and bone health and helps fight allergy problems.[2]

* Grapes and red wines contain protykin, a dietary phytoestrogen. Protykin's unique structure allows for estrogenic and antiestrogenic activities while also providing protective effects for the cardiovascular (heart) system.

* Grapes can help combat cancer, one of the most prevalent—and feared—major illnesses in the United States. Whether seeking to prevent or recover from cancer, grapes or supplements of grape extract can act as part of an effective nutritional approach to overcoming this killer.

* Grapes make a great hunger fighter. When food cravings strike, instead of raiding the fridge after the late-night news or the snack machine at work, you can regulate your blood sugar by snacking on grapes, and such items as cherries, strawberries, apples, carrots, or peanuts.

The Power of Resveratrol

Resveratrol, a health-promoting compound found in grapes, has been shown to increase life span in several species. One of resveratrol's most studied applications involves the prevention of cardiovascular disease. This plant-derived compound appears to act through several different mechanisms to protect the cardiovascular system. Resveratrol may inhibit platelets from clumping together, thus reducing the risk of deadly blood clots that can lead to heart attack and stroke.

How powerful is resveratrol? Consider the mystery surrounding the French, whose cuisine is known for its rich sauces, gourmet cheeses, and fine wines. Why, then, do the French enjoy a relatively low incidence of coronary artery disease? The question may be answered by studies suggesting that it may be the resveratrol, a constituent of the red wine the French drink often. This may have been protecting them from the adverse health effects of their rich diet while also protecting their livers against the toxic effects of alcohol.[3] Could this be a French paradox solved? Just maybe.

Resveratrol's polyphenol is a natural protective agent that makes grapes resilient to attacks by microorganisms. As a rule, resveratrol is in the skins and seeds of the grapes, which are left in much longer during the fermentation process for red wines than for white. Therefore, red wines have higher levels of this valuable compound. Grapes that are grown in harsher climates also seem to have higher levels of resveratrol than those grown in more temperate areas. It seems the more the grapes suffer, the better they are for us.

Since the resveratrol resides in the skins and seeds, it is not as easily absorbed into our bodies in the raw form as when the grapes are crushed and fermented whole into red wine. In fact, the fermentation process for red wine also makes it rich in polyphenols. Red wines are probably the most complex beverages in the human diet because of all the different molecules in them. The bottling process for wines help preserve the resveratrol, while other things that come from grapes, such as raisins, have had almost all of the resveratrol leeched out of them.

Resveratrol was the first natural nutrient to offer significant evidence as a cancer preventative and one that will arrest cancer right in its footsteps. The resveratrol found in grapes and wine (and polyphenols from olive oil) is a promising anticancer agent for both hormone-dependent and hormone-independent breast cancers. It may mitigate the growth stimulatory effect of linoleic acid in the Western-style diet.[4]

Resveratrol has been proven effective in reducing the risk and/or growth of breast, prostate, colon, skin, pancreatic, ovarian, liver, lung, stomach, oral, cervical, lymphatic, thyroid, and esophageal cancers, as well as melanoma, leukemia, metastasis to bones, and neuroblastoma. Research is being done on its ability to boost the effects of chemotherapy and to do its work without harming normal, noncancerous cells. In addition to their anti-carcinogenic properties, phytochemicals like resveratrol have also been reported to bring about a variety of anti-inflammatory and anti-platelet effects.[5]

Healthy Impact

In addition to its cardioprotective effects, resveratrol exhibits a range of anticancer properties. Resveratrol shows promise in protecting our brains and nervous systems against disorders associated with aging and genetic factors. In laboratory studies resveratrol's antioxidant effect has been shown to protect against nerve cell damage caused by beta-amyloid peptide, which accumulates in the brains of Alzheimer's sufferers.

Here's more about this incredible substance: resveratrol may offer benefits in preventing or managing conditions associated with high blood sugar, such as metabolic syndrome or diabetes. Resveratrol is showing promise as a potential therapy for arthritis due to its ability to block the activity of inflammatory compounds. While red wine does contain resveratrol, the quantity varies depending on where the grapes were grown, the time of harvest, and other factors.

Grape and cranberry juices also have resveratrol in them, but contain only about a tenth of the level of red wines—plus they have too much sugar.

The Benefits of Resveratrol

Resveratrol—a compound found in red grapes and red wine—has anti-carcinogenic effects. Resveratrol has the ability to interfere with several processes that are important in the progression of tumors and is very effective in preventing breast, colon, and esophageal cancer.

For those who don't drink or don't care to consume the kind of alcohol necessary to get adequate resveratrol, remember there are supplements. Living Resveratrol can provide you the resveratrol of six hundred glasses of red wine without having to drink any. Such supplements are often extracted from ground-up Japanese knotweed, which is remarkably high in resveratrol.

Despite all the positive aspects of resveratrol in grapes, there is one caution with this delicious fruit. When raised through conventional methods, they are one of the fruits most likely to retain pesticide residues. So, whether choosing grapes or red wine, it is best to choose organic varieties.

For those who don't want the alcohol present in red wines, there are non-alcoholic alternatives you can find in most health food stores. In addition, since drinking enough red wine to derive the optimal health benefits of resveratrol may not be practical or medically advisable, you may want to consider a supplement. A 100 milligram resveratrol capsule per day can provide the protective benefits of this life-extending substance.

Chapter 3

NUTS TO YOU!

SOME PEOPLE SUGGEST saying "nuts" to nuts because they are full of fat. Not true. Nuts are among the foods on a long list of healthy fats. Among those on the long list of beneficial nuts are almonds, walnuts, pistachios, pecans, macadamias, cashews, hickory, soy nuts, Brazil nuts, hazelnuts, and chestnuts. In cooking you can use organic macadamia nut oil for stir-frying at low heat.

The results from a recent study indicate that almond consumption may reduce colon cancer risk via at least one almond lipid-associated component. Such tests show that not all fats are your enemy. Instead, you need to learn to choose good fats and avoid or limit bad fats. Adequate fat intake helps you maintain protein so your body doesn't burn protein as fuel. Fats are also the building blocks for cell membranes.

Instead of snacking on high-caloric, fat-laden, chemical-rich, processed junk food, people living in the Mediterranean region satiate between-meal appetites by eating nuts. This is smart, because studies report that almond consumption may reduce colon cancer risk. Western dieticians, ignorant of the health benefits of nuts, have scared us away from them because of their high fat and caloric content. Nonetheless, almonds and other nuts appear to confer important health benefits.[1]

Studies also show that frequently eating nuts dramatically improves health by significantly lowering the risk of heart disease. A group of researchers at Loma Linda University in California performed a study on 31,000 white Californian Seventh-Day Adventists in 1992. Referred to as the Adventist Health Study, it reported that those persons who ate nuts daily had up to 60 percent fewer heart attacks than those who ate nuts less than once per month.[2] Daily nut consumption benefited everyone in the study, regardless of gender, diet, or physical condition. Benefits were noted as well in another study of African Americans.[3]

Want more proof? It has been calculated that daily nut eaters gain an extra five to six years of life free from coronary artery disease; nut eating appears to increase longevity by about two years.[4] Studies suggest that 1 to 2 ounces of nuts should be consumed daily to gain the maximum benefits from these little "powerhouses" of nutrition. Plus, the protein content of nuts ranges from 10–25 percent, which makes them a great alternative to meat as a source of protein. Because it is plant protein, there is no cholesterol and very little saturated fat involved.

HEALTHY ADVANTAGES

With the exception of those suffering from a peanut allergy, nuts are a healthy carbohydrate that can serve as one of the cornerstones of a sensible weight-loss plan. They will help decrease insulin resistance, which in turn enables you to lose weight. Our bodies need the proper balance of good healthy oils for all our cells, tissues, and organs to function properly. (A caution: you can't expect to gorge on an entire package of cashews, pistachios, or other kinds of nuts and expect positive results. Whatever the food group, moderation is a key.)

While nuts in general are a beneficial part of a healthy diet, walnuts contain almost twice the healthy antioxidants as other nuts. They also contain high amounts of alpha-linolenic acid (ALA), which is associated with lower risk of heart attacks and blood clots. Nutrients in walnuts are also known for their vascular reactivity, or the ability of blood vessels to respond positively to changes in the environment.

Nuts are a good source of magnesium, which is vital for healthy blood pressure and a robust cardiovascular system. This powerful mineral is linked to more than 325 different enzyme reactions in the body. If your body is deficient in magnesium, you could be predisposed to developing hypertension, arrhythmias, and other cardiovascular conditions. This deficiency is one of the most common in the U.S., especially among the elderly. Causes include too much coffee, alcohol, and processed foods.

As mentioned earlier, nuts are a source of plant protein. This is of particular interest to anyone fighting cancer, since cancer patients need adequate protein intake, but not via toxic processed meats— such as bologna, bacon, or sausage—or excessive amounts of red meat or pork. Patients contemplating a snack to stave off hunger until dinnertime will do much better reaching for a handful of raw almonds than candy bars or chips.

RICH IN FIBER

Nuts are full of fiber too, which is one key for the millions of Americans who are battling various forms of diabetes or have prediabetes. Dietary fiber is extremely important in helping to control diabetes. Fiber slows down digestion and the absorption of carbohydrates. This allows for a more gradual rise in blood sugar.

If you have diabetes, a significant amount of the carbohydrate calories you eat should come from vegetables, including peas, beans, lentils, and legumes. Those vegetables typically contain large amounts of fiber. The more soluble fiber in your diet, the better blood sugar control your body will have. Water-soluble fibers are found in nuts as well as oat bran, seeds such as psyllium (the primary ingredient in Metamucil), vegetables, fruit (especially apples and pears), and beans. You should aim to consume at least 30 to 35 grams of fiber a day. You also should take the fiber with meals in order to prevent rapid rises in blood sugar.

Walnuts, almonds, and macadamia nuts are among the sources that can replace unhealthy breads (especially white) and non-nutritious, sugary, and non-whole-grain cereals so many people eat for breakfast. Whether with a meal or as a snack, you can enjoy a tablespoon (about 10) of nuts with no worries about fat. Combined with fresh, low-sugar fruits at breakfast or lunch and such items as steamed, stir-fried, or raw vegetables, lean meats, and salads with colorful vegetables, nuts are a vital element of a healthy eating plan.

Nuts: B the One

In addition to such benefits as their fiber and healthy oils, nuts are a nutritious source of healthy B vitamins, including:

- Riboflavin (vitamin B_2), which helps body cells create energy from carbohydrates, protein, and fat. It is crucial for normal growth and repair and tissue development.
- Niacin (also known as B_3), which assists in the functioning of your digestive system and keeps skin and nerves healthy. Niacin is important for the conversion of food to energy.
- Vitamin B_6 refers to a group of water soluble vitamins that help maintain healthy brain and nerve functions, fight diseases, form red blood cells, and digest proteins.

OTHER HEALTH BENEFITS

There are other reasons to eat nuts. They contain potassium, a healthy mineral that is in short supply in the standard Western diet. And nuts, such as pecans, cashews, and pine nuts, are rich in zinc, which is necessary for the proper functioning of several enzymatic functions that are important for healthy skin. Zinc also promotes cell division, repair, and growth. It helps the lymphatic system to oxygenate the tissues and eliminate wastes properly. And it works synergistically with other minerals and vitamins. For instance, in combination with sulfur and vitamin A, zinc helps to build strong hair.

In addition, nuts contain essential omega-3 fatty acids; these acids are fantastic disease fighters. Several thousand scientific publications testify to widespread agreement among medical professionals about the benefits of omega-3 fatty acids. For years doctors have recognized the benefits of the Mediterranean diet, which is rich in omega-3 fatty acids. Studies show that individuals who get a sufficient amount of omega-3 fatty acids in their diets experience a significantly lower risk of cancer mortality.

Some of the best sources of these acids are plants, along with fish and oils. Plants and oils contain the acid known as ALA (alpha-linolenic acid). Plant sources relatively high in ALA content include nuts, seeds, and soybeans. Fish are high in the omega-3 acids known as ALA, eicosapentaenoic acid (EPA), and docosahexaenoic acid (DHA).

Chapter 4

CELERY: POWERFUL HEALER

THE MODEST CELERY stick can be found on many dining room tables, hors d'oeuvre trays, and snack carts. Yet its healing and protective powers have rightfully earned it a place on the superfoods list. As an example, celery and such powerhouses as garlic, wild salmon, walnuts, and dark chocolate are leaders in improving heart health and lowering blood pressure.

One of the most dramatic stories about celery appears in the most recent edition of the book, *The New Healing Herbs*. It concerns Mr. Minh Le, who ate four celery stalks for one week and took three weeks off to help lower his high blood pressure. Mr. Le saw his blood pressure drop from 158/96 to 118/82 within one week!

By way of his son, Minh Le brought awareness of this ancient Chinese remedy to researchers at the University of Chicago Medical Center. The investigators tested animals by injecting the mammals with a small amount of 3-n-butylphthalide, a chemical compound that is found in celery. Mr. Minh Le's son, Quang Le, and University of Chicago pharmacologist William Elliot, PhD, isolated the compound 3-n-butylphthalide and injected rats with the equivalent amount of what's found in four stalks of celery.

Not only did the rats' blood pressure drop 13 percent in a week, their cholesterol levels also dropped by 7 percent. The chemical that reduced the animals' blood pressure readings turned out to be phthalide. It's known in scientific circles that phthalide relaxes the muscles and arteries that regulate blood pressure. Phthalide is a chemical that also reduced the amount of "stress hormones," called catecholamines. Stress hormones also raise blood pressure since catecholamines constrict blood vessels.

These tests gave more validity to celery's reputation as a traditional Asian folk remedy for high blood pressure. However, it is possible that celery may work only if your high blood pressure is caused by too much renin in your blood. (Renin is produced by your kidneys.) If your blood pressure is high because of elevated renin levels and you are given a diuretic for your initial treatment, this could make your blood pressure soar even higher. Find out first if the high blood pressure is caused by too much renin, then consider making celery a part of a high blood pressure treatment plan.

Green Healer

One stalk of celery contains about 35 milligrams of sodium, which should not raise your blood pressure. Be sure to choose organic celery, though. Though a healthy vegetable, traditionally-grown celery is typically high in pesticide residue.[1]

However, its phytonutrients make it stand out as a heart-healthy food. Many of these phytonutrients fall into the category of phenolic antioxidants and have been shown to provide anti-inflammatory benefits as well.[2]

One of the phytonutrients in celery is low concentrations of apigenin. Apigenin inhibits angiogenesis in ovarian cancer cells, which is the process by which tumors instruct the body to build new blood vessels to reach to wherever they happen to have latched on to an organ so that they can feed themselves. Preventing angiogenesis keeps the cancer cells from hijacking the body's food supply for itself and stymies its growth and ability to spread. Apigenin interferes with cancer cells' ability to burn glucose in the pancreas, another important function that starves cancers. Apigenin is also an anti-inflammatory agent. As if that weren't enough, it also promotes apoptosis *within* tumors, shrinking them and heading others off before they even have a chance to form. A 2009 study from Harvard's Channing Laboratory found that of five different flavonoids, only apigenin was associated with a significant reduction in cancer risk.[3]

Celery can fight diabetes problems too. Gabriel Cousens, MD, author of *There Is a Cure for Diabetes*, recommends a series of foods for their therapeutic properties in the treatment of diabetes. One is celery, which has general antidiabetogenic qualities and also helps lower your blood pressure, which is a symptom of metabolic syndrome. Among others are Jerusalem artichoke, cucumbers, garlic, onions, walnuts, almonds, and kelp.[4]

SKIN CLEANSER

Celery is especially great for your skin. It can clean the cells, remove dirt and oil from skin, and can help fight against acne and dilute acne scarring. It is extremely efficient for people who want to lose weight and maintain their health. The exceptional benefits of celery have been recognized for centuries by ancient medical practitioners. Hippocrates, known as the father of modern medicine, claimed that celery played a major role in calming the nerves.[5] The 1897 Sears catalog even offered a nerve tonic made from celery.[6] Celery neutralizes acidity, promotes the proper functioning of the immune system, purifies our bodies, and keeps them in balance.

Furthermore, it is a great source of calcium, which helps to build strong teeth and bones. Celery provides your body with vitamin A and is a great source of B vitamins, such as B_1, B_2, and B_6. The latter give you energy for a fresh start to the day. It is also high in such nutrients as magnesium, iron, folic acid, and potassium.[7] It contains plenty of water too, which provides proper hydration for blood cells. Due to its high water and potassium content, celery is used for cosmetic purposes and is highly effective for treating dry, dehydrated skin.[8] Celery rehydrates the body and helps to maintain a healthy libido.[9]

A Recipe for Clear Skin

Often the secret to clear skin is perfecting your diet. Certain foods are better for your complexion than others, so make sure you incorporate plenty of skin-clearing ingredients into your daily diet. Try out this salad recipe that combines four essential foods for clear skin!

Super Skin Complexion Salad

How to make it: combine lettuce, cucumbers, celery, and papayas. Optional: avocado for added taste and a sense of fullness.

Why it's great for your skin: Celery cleans the skin cells of dirt and removes skin oils, fights acne, and reduces scars. Cucumbers hydrate your skin due to their high water and silica content, which greatly enhances skin tone. Papayas not only taste great, but they also enhance skin beauty due to their high collagen and vitamin C content. Finally, avocados reduce wrinkles and create a more toned skin due to high collagen production from their healthy oils.

THE POWER OF JUICING

Celery is a must as one of the ingredients in creating fresh vegetable juices for your diet. As an example of what it can do, you can attack arthritis problems with a mixture of celery, grapefruit, carrot, and spinach; or carrots and celery. One suggested juice combination to combat gallstones is celery, carrot, and parsley. While fruit juices are wonder cleansers for your body's systems, and they are OK occasionally, they contain a lot of sugar. Vegetable juices are low in sugar and better nutritionally because they have a higher alkaline content than fruit juices, which tend to be acidic. (It is OK to add an apple to vegetable juice to sweeten it, though.)

Therapeutic Celery

Among fresh vegetable juice recipes that use celery and have therapeutic properties:

- For arthritis, try celery juice or a mixture of grapefruit juice, carrot, and spinach juice.
- For nervous tension, try mixing carrot and celery juice.
- For headaches, try a parsley, spinach, celery, and carrot juice combination.

Juices are some of the most powerful whole foods you can put into your body. They can help prevent cancer and heart disease, boost immunity, lower your risk of Alzheimer's disease, and cleanse your body of toxins. They take little effort to digest, so you can benefit almost instantly from their energy and nutrients. Your body absorbs nutrients from juices better than it does from the foods themselves because you break down the plant's cellulose, which makes all of the health-promoting vitamins, minerals, and other healing compounds easier to absorb. Juicing offers the added benefit of weight control, since they leave you feeling satisfied, which helps limit excessive food intake.

While vegetables juices are preferable, both fruit and vegetable juices and a strict regimen of vegetables (no meat) are among nutritional approaches to preventing or recovering from cancer. Drinking at least one pint of juice each day is helpful in the case of other major disorders. Fruit juices are the cleansers of our bodies, and vegetable juices are the builders and regenerators of our systems. Vegetable juices contain all the minerals, salts, amino acids, enzymes, and vitamins that the human body requires.

Chapter 5

SPROUTING HEALTH

NO MATTER HOW many times Grandma counseled you to eat your brussels sprouts, you likely resisted her advice. Let's face it: whether it's brussels sprouts, broccoli, cauliflower, or those strange-looking, stringy things sitting at the end of the salad bar, sprouts aren't likely to make many favorite foods lists. However, while you may not have to be too fond of them, sprouts are a health powerhouse. Because of the different compounds found in broccoli, cauliflower, watercress, cabbage, kale, brussels sprouts, and the like, they have long been among the leading cancer-fighting foods.

Epidemiologic and animal studies have associated certain plants with pronounced reductions in cancer risk. What characteristics of these sprouted vegetables might protect against carcinogenesis? They contain little fat, are low in energy, and are good sources of vitamins, minerals, and fiber—all linked to cancer protection. Some of their phytochemicals protected against carcinogenesis in various tests. Recent research results also show that consumption of cruciferous vegetables, particularly broccoli, plays an important role in decreasing the risk of breast cancer in premenopausal women.

Still not convinced? There is a reason Ezekiel 4:9 bread is one of the healthiest loaves you can find at the market: it comes from the sprouts of wheat, barley, and other grains. For more proof, consider that juices made with such ingredients as sprouts, wheatgrass, barley grass, oat grass, and blue-green algae are wonderful for reversing acidity in the body and are high in chlorophyll. Chlorophyll has been found to have anticancer effects since it protects DNA from damaging radiation.

These foods have also been shown to have antiviral, antitumor, and anti-inflammatory properties. In effect, such foods can actually inhibit carcinogens in cooked meats and even in cigarette smoke. A chlorophyll drink containing one or more of these potent power foods is a good idea, although if you have a high serum iron or ferritin level, you may need to limit intake of green foods.

BROCCOLI BOOST

If green foods aren't a problem, you can't do much better than eating plenty of broccoli, which contains lots of fiber, vitamin C, and antioxidants. In the battle against cancer broccoli's phytohormones, or phytoestrogens, protect the body from carcinogenic mutations. Typically, diets that contain good amounts of these and other phytoestrogen-rich foods help fight against disease.

Broccoli sprouts are high in sulforaphane, which contributes to the detoxification of carcinogens, promotes apoptosis, interrupts cancer cell replication, makes healthy tissue more tumor resistant, fights metastasis, and blocks the cancer-producing effects of exposure to ultraviolet radiation. According to Johns Hopkins University's Paul Talalay, "Three-day-old broccoli sprouts consistently contain 20 to 50 times the amount of chemoprotective compounds found in mature broccoli heads, and may offer a simple, dietary means of chemically reducing cancer risk."[1] These sprouts (or teas made from them) appear to be especially high in these cancer-defeating compounds.

Clover and alfalfa sprouts are also high in phytoestrogens, which are important in preventing breast and prostate cancers. Alfalfa sprouts and wheat sprouts contain both antioxidants and phytonutrients. It appears that "sprouting" these vegetables gives them increased benefits because many of their phytonutrients are potent in the seeds that are only a few days old. Wheat sprouts are high in chlorophyll and also contain chlorophyllin, a powerful phytonutrient. The latter blocks aflatoxin, a carcinogenic fungus that grows on grains such as corn and rice. It also blocks heterocyclic amines, which are carcinogenic.

To add to the positive picture of alfalfa, it contains large amounts of chlorophyll, beta-carotene, and vitamin E. Alfalfa contains the nonprotein amino acid L-canavanine, which has antibacterial, antiviral, and antitumoral activities. L-canavanine inhibited the in vitro growth of human pancreatic cancer and human melanoma. This nonprotein amino acid sensitized human colon and pancreatic cancer cells to Y-irradiation and enhanced the effect of 5-fluorouracil. It has also been shown that L-canavanine's antitumor mechanism of action is growth inhibition. Certain studies also indicate that L-canavanine, in combination with radiation, could have clinical potential in the treatment of cancer.

As one expert in the field, Gabriel Cousens, put it, "Sprouts contain a rainforest of undiscovered and known good health characteristics such as antioxidants, anti-carcinogens, live enzymes, high levels of vitamins, nucleic acids, paciferans (plant antibiotics), auxones (beneficial plant hormones), and other factors."[2]

CHROMIUM-RICH FOODS

There are other reasons to eat healthy servings of sprouts, starting with chromium, which is found in broccoli, grapefruit, and fortified breakfast cereals. This mineral helps to regulate blood and keep it in balance, according to Richard A. Anderson, PhD, a research chemist with the USDA Human Nutrition Research Council in Beltsville, Maryland.[3] Chromium metabolizes amino acids and fats and helps to lower bad cholesterol while raising the good.

Elevated blood sugar spurs the body to secrete insulin; chronically high insulin levels can lead to obesity, high blood pressure, and high triglycerides. All of these reactions boost the risk of heart disease. As we get older, our bodies store less chromium, which may account for the reason age is one of the biggest risk factors in the development of diabetes. Therefore, this wonderful mineral is useful for controlling diabetes and hypoglycemia as well as preventing cardiovascular disease.

Tests show that people with diabetes have lower levels of chromium circulating in their blood than people without the disease. In one study eight participants who had difficulty regulating blood sugar took 200 micrograms (mcg.) of chromium per day. After five weeks their blood sugar levels fell by as much as 50 percent. People without blood sugar problems who took chromium showed no such changes.[4] So in essence, chromium offers you "chrome-plated" protection.

Chromium is a difficult mineral to absorb, and most of it is eliminated through the kidneys and bowels. Complex carbohydrates can help your body retain chromium, while sugary foods will cause your body to excrete chromium. If that weren't bad enough, sugary foods contribute to diabetes, obesity, and other health problems.

Making Up Deficiencies

Sprouts can help your body make up for deficiencies, such as shortages in magnesium, an important mineral required for energy production, processing sugar, and other tasks, such as contributing to the development of healthy bones. Magnesium also assists with the active transport of calcium and potassium ions across cell membranes, a process that is vital to nerve impulse conduction, muscle contraction, and normal heart rhythm.[5]

Broccoli is one of the many foods that increase GABA levels, as do almonds, tree nuts, bananas, lentils, and brown rice. GABA is a chemical in the brain that helps you relax, reduces anxiety and stress, and increases alertness. And it keeps all the other neurotransmitters and hormones in check. People with a GABA deficiency can become irritable, experience chronic anxiety, and have difficulty handling life's day-to-day stresses. Among other symptoms are headaches, heart disorders, and high blood pressure.

Sprouts help your body get more B vitamins too. Broccoli and vegetables in the cabbage family will help you get more vitamin B_5 from food, while bean sprouts are among foods that provide vitamin B_9. More widely known as folate, B_9 has many longevity-promoting benefits, including protection from cardiovascular disease.

Choose Fresh

A final word on the sprouts that pack such power: search for fresh sources. Because of consumer demand for good-looking produce, the food industry seeks to protect fragile vegetables and fruits through special packaging. But good appearance can't hide the fact that when picked and left outside more than two or three hours, their nutritional value declines dramatically. Spinach greens, asparagus, broccoli, and peas lose 50 percent of their vitamins before they ever get to market. Packaging and transporting produce compromises nutritional values even more, as does produce sitting in storage.

To increase shelf life and appearance, farmers harvest fruits and vegetables long before they are mature. That might seem innocent enough, but fruits and vegetables absorb most of their vitamins and minerals when they are almost ripe. Remember, that bunch of bright green bananas will never fill up with the vitamins and minerals they would have acquired ripening in the sun instead of sitting on the shelf. If you can grow your own sprouted veggies or have access to a farmer's market, your bottom line will look much healthier.

Chapter 6

GO FOR GARLIC

O NE OF NATURE'S most potent antibiotics garlic is a shining example of a superfood whose benefits read like a "Who's Who" of good health. Among its benefits:

+ Improves heart health
+ Lowers blood pressure
+ Inhibits the growth of fungi, yeast, and bacteria, including strains that are becoming resistant to synthetic antibiotics
+ Boosts the immune system, which helps prevent colds
+ Improves detoxification
+ Contains antioxidant properties
+ Contains sulfur compounds that are believed to be the reason for its anti-diabetic effects
+ Works as an anti-inflammatory substance. This is particularly significant when it comes to America, where the toxic state of the standard American diet produces significantly more heart disease.

The healing potential of this pungent bulb has been recognized for thousands of years. It was prescribed by legendary, fifth-century Greek physician Hippocrates as a cure-all in an ancient Sanskrit manuscript. Throughout history garlic has been used to treat everything from wounds and infections to digestive complaints. During World War II, when Russians ran out of penicillin for their battle wounds, they requisitioned garlic cloves, which is where garlic got its famous nickname "Russian penicillin."

Established Curative Agent

More than one thousand research papers have established the chemistry and pharmacology of garlic. Garlic is used for many conditions related to the heart and circulatory system, including high blood pressure, high cholesterol, coronary heart disease, heart attack, and hardening of the arteries (atherosclerosis). Studies have shown that garlic is effective in slowing the development of atherosclerosis and reducing blood pressure.

Recent reports by the National Cancer Institute on a large population of subjects in China indicate that the consumption of garlic and other members of the allium genus (onions, leeks, and shallots) may help lower the incidence of stomach cancer.[1] Here's why. Allicin, the active ingredient in garlic, is a compound that works like aspirin to thin the blood, which helps prevent atherosclerosis and coronary blockages. It helps lower cholesterol, reduce blood clot formation, prevent yeast overgrowth, stimulate the pituitary, regulate blood sugar, and prevent cancer, particularly in the gastrointestinal tract. In addition, it is antibacterial, antifungal, and may often be used to treat minor infections.

Not Just for Spaghetti

Get the best garlic has to offer by:

- Enjoying it fresh: Crushed garlic contains allicin, a compound that breaks down into a cascade of healthful compounds.
- Eating for convenience: Raw, cooked, powdered—the choice is yours. All forms have their benefits!
- Cutting it fine: Whether cooked or eaten raw, mincing, crushing, or pressing garlic will vastly

> expand its surface area and give you the maximum number of healthful compounds.
>
> - Taking it as a liquid extract: You will find it at your local health food store. Just follow the label directions. Or, take one to two capsules of an aged garlic product daily.

Furthermore, garlic contains at least twenty-five germ-killing compounds and fights off bacterial, fungal, and even viral infections. It has been shown to have the ability to aid certain immune functions, particularly increasing the activity of natural killer cells.[2] Such benefits aren't seen only in the laboratory. People in southern Italy who eat a lot of garlic develop less stomach cancer than those Italians who live in the north (who typically do not eat much, if any, garlic).

Despite this myriad of benefits, in order for garlic to be effective in reversing heart conditions, it must have the right amount of allicin. Since odorless garlic supplements reduce the amount of allicin, this compromises the product's effectiveness. Methods that involve crushing the fresh clove release more allicin.[3]

CANCER FIGHTER

Garlic (and onions) contains phytochemical compounds that appear particularly good at keeping the nitrates and nitrites in our foods from converting into nitrosamines, a class of compounds with numerous cancer-causing characteristics. Because of this, garlic (and onions) seems particularly effective in preventing esophageal, stomach, and colon cancers. Nitrates are particularly high in pickled foods and processed or cured meats such as sausage, bacon, and ham. While vegetables also contain some nitrates, these seem to be counteracted by the vitamin C they also contain; thus these plant nitrates do not turn into toxic compounds. While garlic appears to have a greater protective power than onions, the latter are far more prevalent in most Western diets. Crushed fresh garlic seems to have the highest amount of cancer-fighting compounds.

Besides these preventative qualities, molecules found in these vegetables also appear to slow the spread of tumors and encourage apoptosis through interfering with the growth process of cancer cells. While more study is needed to determine how exactly compounds in garlic and onions have these effects, there is enough evidence now available to suggest that adding these allium family vegetables to spice up our foods is a wise step toward an anticancer diet plan.

Several years ago noted cancer surgeon Francesco Contreras, who has gained international attention both for his skills and ability to integrate natural therapies with orthodox medicine, started using Kyolic Aged Garlic Extract as a natural antibiotic to treat ear infections. He first observed it working wonders with his children. Later it earned a permanent spot in his medical treatments when he discovered its effectiveness as an anti-stress and anti-fatigue agent. When research demonstrated the role garlic plays in the health of the heart, a question occurred to him: Could garlic offer similar benefits to cancer patients and people wishing to avoid it?

The Best Medicine

Garlic can do more than make flavorful spaghetti. For example:

- For a rapid immune system fix, try two cloves of garlic and one slice of ginger. Garlic and ginger are natural antibiotics that boost a weakened immune system.

- Ever get struck by a toothache while traveling? Instead of suffering through sleepless nights, try this natural remedy for toothaches: chew on a clove

of garlic. A natural antibiotic, garlic kills bacteria
and, in most cases, works as good as a painkiller.

SLOWING TUMORS' DEVELOPMENT

When he reviewed the medical literature, Contreras was thrilled
to find that aged garlic extract constituents have been shown to
be effective in inhibiting the growth and development of prostate
cancer cells, melanoma cells, and neuroblastoma cells. In addition
these constituents slow the growth and development of carcinogen-
induced tumors of the bladder, breast, colon, esophagus, stomach,
and lung.

Dr. Contreras was impressed with the extensive nature of
these clinical studies. G. Li and collaborators found that two ele-
ments in aged garlic extract, called S-allyl cysteine (SAC) and
S-allyl-mercaptocysteine, inhibit the growth and proliferation of
breast cancer cells.[4] Even better, they equip surrounding cells with
tools they desperately need, such as gluthathione-S-transferase
and peroxidase. These are critical agents in cell detoxification
and gene expression. In other words, they help cells get rid of the
toxins that damage their ability to reproduce properly. When the
gene expression process is compromised, the result is often a can-
cerous cell. Much of garlic's activity derives from aliin and allicin
or its immediate byproducts, such as S-allyl cysteine and S-allyl-
mercaptocysteine. Garlic also contains selenium and tellurium.

Among aged garlic's other extract attributes are its anti-infection,
anti-aging, cardioprotective, and immune-enhancement properties.
Additional research suggests that aged garlic extract might be useful
for treating physiological aging and age-related memory disorders in
humans. While not claiming that garlic can cure cancer, the physician says that the constituents in aged garlic extract are important

in combating carcinogens within the body. "Clearly, garlic and aged garlic extract should be an integral part of your effort to equip your body to ward off disease," Dr. Contreras says, noting a study conducted at Tufts University School of Medicine in Boston. It concluded that aged garlic extract actually protects healthy cells against the oxidizing damage caused by chemotherapy.[5]

Helping the Liver

Garlic has another impressive quality. It is a natural liver-supporting food that can aid the liver in detoxifying itself naturally—as do such foods as grapefruit, green vegetables, avocados, walnuts, the spice turmeric, and green tea. These foods help the liver produce enzymes and amino acids that help the liver rid itself of the toxins it encounters daily. Most people have a clogged or sluggish liver, which can lead to things such as metabolism slowing as fat stores increase, digestion slowing down, and appetite and food cravings increasing. Detoxifying the liver is key to good health, since once it is cleansed other organs will follow suit.

Chapter 7

MIGHTY MUSHROOMS

I T's TIME FOR Americans to learn what the Chinese and Japanese have known for generations: mushrooms are packed with power. Not only are they important sources of nutrients that stimulate the immune system, but researchers say that mushrooms also possibly help fight cancer, high cholesterol, and perhaps even the AIDS virus. They boost immune function, lower bad cholesterol, regulate blood sugar, and protect your body from viruses and possibly cancer by inhibiting tumor growth. They contain bioactive molecules and essential amino acids, and feature a low fat content.

For three thousand years Asians have enjoyed the power of mushrooms, both for their taste and therapeutic value. In fact, Chinese legend is filled with stories of people who discovered a one-thousand-year-old mushroom and became immortal! This is a little far-fetched. However, while mushrooms cannot promise immortality, they do provide polysaccharides, sterols, coumarin, vitamins, minerals, and amino acids.

Today there are about thirty-five different species of mushrooms to partake of; most are edible and have medicinal properties. Scientists are now discovering what natural healers have known for centuries. One of particular note is the reishi mushroom, which lately has received considerable attention for its apparent immune-enhancing activities; this may confirm the wisdom of traditional Chinese medical practitioners, who have used them for centuries.

Studies have shown that reishi may transform many components of the immune system, including natural killer cells. Moreover, one study concluded that reishi's effect on such immune-related cells as

T and B cells yielded further evidence that reishi's value comes from its ability to enhance immunity response.[1]

In the past America's favorite mushroom, "the button," was never thought to have much medicinal value, but recent studies have found that this little mushroom packs quite a punch when it comes to preventing breast cancer. [2] Other forms of mushrooms were also found to help prevent breast cancer. White stuffing mushrooms offered the strongest amount of protection, followed by shiitake, portobello, cremini, and baby button. All of these mushrooms showed a significant effect, whether eaten raw or cooked.

Recipe: Asparagus and Mushroom Pasta

1 lb. thin asparagus

3/4 lb. mushrooms (use your favorite)

1 Tbsp. extra-virgin olive oil

1/4 cup dry white wine

1/2 cup vegetable broth

4 Tbsp. unsalted butter

Sea salt and freshly ground black pepper

Fettuccine

1 Tbsp. flat leaf parsley

Cut off the tough ends of the asparagus and mushrooms and slice them into bite-size pieces. In a large skillet, heat the oil over medium high heat; add mushrooms and cook, stirring until lightly browned. Add the asparagus and cook, stirring for two minutes. Add the wine and simmer until the liquid is evaporated. Add the vegetable broth and bring to a boil. Add the butter and toss until melted into the veggies. Season to taste.

> In a large pot of boiling, salted water, cook pasta according to directions. Drain and transfer to a large bowl. Mix in the sauce and the parsley. Season to taste with additional salt and pepper.

Although raw mushrooms are a favorite at most salad bars, do not make a habit of eating the uncooked kind. Raw mushrooms contain hydrazines, which are toxic chemicals. Since no one is sure of just how many raw mushrooms you would have to eat in order to enter a "danger zone," it is better to cook all of your mushrooms, since the heating process eliminates hydrazines. Besides, for both taste and nutrition, mushrooms are better cooked. This is because they are mostly water. Cooking not only removes the water, it also concentrates the nutrients and the flavor.

In addition to maitake, shiitake, and reishi, you may want to try oyster, morel, porcini, cremini, and portobello. All of these mushrooms offer you far-reaching health benefits. You can add them to vegetables, soups, casseroles, or stir-fry dishes.

THE AGING PROCESS

The simple process of aging depletes your storehouse of nucleic acids, which are the building blocks of DNA and RNA. These two substances are present in each cell of your body. Exposure to chemicals, harsh environmental factors, and lower levels of protective phytonutrients in the diet make it important to support healthy function of DNA in our bodies. Proper function of our DNA code—imprinted in all nucleated cells of our body—and proper function of our immune system may well be the two most critical factors involved in maintaining health. The major function of DNA, beyond carrying the genetic traits of our ancestors, is to duplicate itself exactly when cells divide.

It is crucial to protect DNA in order to continually synthesize perfect copies of complex proteins called enzymes in order to maintain healthy metabolism and cellular functions.[3] DNA maintenance enzymes within the cells are responsible for ensuring that the code remains the same when a cell divides, accomplishing this before, during, or after cell division. Your body ensures cellular health through a process called apoptosis. During apoptosis, cells that are unable to maintain accurate DNA copies through their own DNA repair mechanisms are broken down and recycled. The body has numerous such processes to maintain and promote healthy DNA, which results in healthy cells, including a healthy immune system.

The Healthy Mushroom

Mushrooms are good for helping replenish your stock of nucleic acids, which may:

- Slow the aging process
- Increase energy
- Promote healthier skin and reduce age spots

In addition to spinach, some other nucleic-rich foods are salmon, wheat germ, and asparagus. You also add a B-complex vitamin to increase these acids.

Protecting DNA keeps aging at bay. To protect and promote healthy DNA, it is important to know that vitamin B_{12} and folic acid play a role in methylation reactions, which are essential to maintaining healthy DNA. In addition, vitamins B_{12}, B_9 (folic acid), B_8 (biotin), and B_6 (pyridoxine) promote cell longevity, DNA and RNA production, nucleic acid formation, and RNA/DNA action. Mushrooms are a rich food source of nucleic acids, as are spinach, asparagus, salmon, and wheat germ.

BALANCING YOUR BRAIN

Mushrooms are one of the "brain foods" that you can work into your diet to help improve nutritional balance. That equals body balance, which equals brain balance. Your body uses the nutrition with which you supply it to build, maintain, and repair your tissues. Nutrients empower your cells to relay messages back and forth to conduct essential chemical reactions that enable you to think, see, hear, smell, taste, move, breathe, and eliminate waste.

Human beings share the same basic physical makeup, but each of us is as individual as our thumbprint when it comes to our specific nutritional needs. Many factors combine to determine your individual nutritional needs, including the amount of stress you face and how you manage it, whether you live a hectic lifestyle that depletes your nutritional storehouse, dietary habits, and whether you are overly acidic or overly alkaline.

The latter terms refer to the composition of our bodies. In childhood most people are naturally alkaline, which is true into the teen years and early adulthood. But by the fourth decade of life, most people become overly acidic because of exposure to stress, poor food selections, and environmental toxins. Being overly acidic makes the body susceptible to many ailments, including headaches, chronic illnesses, colds and flu, digestive problems, urinary tract infections, and chronic fatigue. Having a healthy acid/alkaline balance means enjoying better mental clarity, fast recovery from illness and injury, vitality, and energy. The good news is that you can bring your system into a more balanced state by eating foods that will turn acidic conditions around.

There is a long list of foods that should become part of your dietary regimen. In addition to mushrooms, among other vegetables that contribute to healthy balance are sweet peppers, spinach, carrots, squash, asparagus, onions, peas, celery, and lettuce. So do such things as legumes (baked beans, kidney beans, lima beans, black beans), grains such as brown rice and barley, free-range chicken eggs, tofu, unsweetened (not canned) fruits, and nuts and seeds.

If you are overly acidic, you will feel better if you consume more complex carbohydrates in your daily diet. If you are a high alkaline producer, you will feel better if your diet contains more proteins. Complex carbohydrates mean a combination of whole grains and legumes. When it comes to protein, fish and poultry are better than red meats for both metabolic types because they are lower in unhealthy saturated fat, and they contain a full spectrum of essential amino acids, as well as being great sources of vitamins E, D, and A.

Chapter 8

SPINACH: POPEYE KNEW HIS STUFF

CARTOON AFICIONADOS KNOW that Popeye made himself super strong by eating spinach, but the power of this dark green, leafy vegetable is not a myth. Spinach offers real-life protection against osteoporosis, heart disease, colon cancer, arthritis, and other diseases. And it contains heart-healthy vitamins, minerals, and antioxidants. These nutrients help reduce the risk of heart disease, which is why spinach and such greens as kale, collards, turnip, and mustard rank among the top anti-inflammatory foods.

Eating spinach also supplies you with antioxidants, vitamins B_6 and B_{12}, and flavonoids. Researchers have identified at least thirteen different flavonoid compounds in spinach that function as antioxidants and as anticancer agents. The anticancer properties of these spinach flavonoids have been shown to slow cell division in stomach cancer cells and to reduce skin cancers. A study on adult women living in New England in the late 1980s also showed intake of spinach to be inversely related to incidence of breast cancer.

What's more, spinach is high in folate. Folate helps reduce homocysteine, a toxic amino acid that accelerates plaque formation and is usually a by-product from consuming meat. When homocysteine is present in high levels in the blood, it is associated with hardening and narrowing of the arteries, increased risk of heart attack, stroke, and blood clots.

Spinach's high levels of folate and vitamin B_{12} may also protect the brain against dementia. Researchers from Tufts and Boston Universities observed subjects in the Framingham Heart Study and found those with high levels of homocysteine had nearly double the risk of developing Alzheimer's disease. High homocysteine is associated with low levels of folate and vitamins B_6 and B_{12}, leading researchers to speculate that getting more B vitamins may be protective. It appears that high homocysteine levels can be reduced safely by adding modest amounts of folate to your diet.

Recipe: Popeye's Favorite Stir-fry

1 lb. beef eye of round

1 Tbsp. cornstarch

1 tsp. canola oil

2 tsp. grated fresh ginger

1 small onion, thinly sliced

1 bag (6 oz.) spinach, washed and trimmed

1/3 cup defatted beef broth

2 Tbsp. ketchup

Black pepper and sea salt, to taste

Cut the beef across the grain into very thin slices. Place in a medium bowl. Add cornstarch and toss to coat.

In a wok or large skillet, heat oil over medium high heat until it is nearly smoking. Add the beef and ginger. Stir-fry until the beef is no longer pink on the surface, about two minutes. Transfer to a plate.

Add the onion to the pan, and stir-fry until softened, one to two minutes. Add the spinach and stir-fry until just wilted, about thirty seconds.

In a small bowl, combine the broth and ketchup. Add to the pan. Add the beef. Stir-fry until the sauce is heated through and coats the beef and vegetables, about two to three minutes.

Season to taste with sea salt and pepper. Serve over brown rice! Makes four servings, containing 207 calories each.

LONGEVITY BENEFITS

Folate has many longevity-promoting benefits as well. Studies have shown that people with the most folate in their blood are the ones least likely to develop colon cancer, particularly cigarette smokers, as reported by the Karolinska Institute in Sweden and the Harvard School of Public Health.[1]

To clarify the possible influence of smoking on folate's protective effect against colon cancer, the study followed more than sixty-one thousand women. Using food frequency questionnaires, the researchers determined mean daily folate intake among the study subjects at 183 mcg. During nearly fifteen years of follow-up, researchers documented 805 cases of colorectal cancer in the study group. Women who ingested less than 150 mcg. of folate daily had a 39 percent greater risk of colon cancer, compared to women who consumed at least 212 mcg. Researchers observed a dose-related response relationship between daily folate intake and colon cancer risk, predicting that each 100-mcg. increase in folate intake could decrease colon cancer risk by 34 percent.

Among women who had smoked cigarettes for ten or more years, those consuming at least 193 mcg. of folate daily had a 66 percent lower risk of colon cancer than those whose intake was less than 163 mcg. Although nonsmokers with the lowest folate intake had a 41 percent lower risk of colon cancer than did smokers, smokers with the highest folate intake had the same risk of colon cancer as non-smokers with the highest folate intake.

What this means to the average person is that increasing dietary folate intake may decrease the risk of colon cancer. This is especially notable in smokers, who experience an elevated risk for the disease. In addition, studies are now pointing to possible connections between folate intake and the risk of cognitive problems, particularly Alzheimer's disease.[2]

THE GLYCEMIC ADVANTAGE

Spinach is full of fiber, an essential component of a healthy diet. To get adequate fiber, experts recommend eating at least five servings of vegetables and fruit daily. In addition to spinach, other fiber-filled veggies are peas, broccoli, raw carrots, parsnips, and brussels sprouts.

Vegetables are particularly noted for their low values on the glycemic index, which we briefly mentioned in chapter 5 on sprouts.

This index is a scale that measures how the body processes various foods. However, the healthy advantage of vegetables did not automatically extend to all low-index foods. Almost twenty years after the creation of the glycemic index, researchers at Harvard University developed an updated method for classifying foods. It took into account not only their glycemic index value but also their quantity of carbohydrates. They named this more comprehensive scale the glycemic load (GL). It serves as a guide as to how much of a particular carbohydrate or food people should eat.

The reason for the revision? For a while nutritionists scratched their heads over patients who wanted to lose weight and were eating low-glycemic foods, yet many weren't shedding pounds; some gained weight. The GL revealed that overconsuming many low-glycemic foods can cause weight gain. Not surprisingly many patients were eating as many low-glycemic foods as they wanted, simply because they thought that foods with a low value promoted weight loss. Such would-be dieters needed to know the whole story. The glycemic load balanced the picture. A food's GL is determined by multiplying the glycemic index value by the quantity of carbohydrates a serving contains (in grams), and then dividing that number by 100. The formula looks like this:

(Glycemic Index Value x Carb Grams per Serving) ÷ 100 = Glycemic Load

To demonstrate the value of the GL, some wheat pastas have a low glycemic index value. That makes many dieters think they're a key to losing weight. However, overly large serving sizes can sabotage weight loss. Despite a low glycemic index value, the pasta's GL is high. Another example is white potatoes, whose GL is double that of yams. The amount of fiber, fat, and proteins in your food and how much sugar is in the carbohydrates all determine the new glycemic index score of what you eat.

Even with this revision, spinach comes out smelling like a rose, with a rating of 15 (on a scale of 1 to 100) of 15. So does asparagus, celery, broccoli, cucumbers, green beans, all varieties of peppers, and low fat yogurt.[3]

JUICING AND BLENDING

Spinach is as good for you raw as it is cooked, and even better when tossed into a juicer or blender. Using a juicer or blender sends natural nutrients and raw energy straight into your bloodstream. Freshly juiced fruits and vegetables are better for you. Unlike more time-consuming raw fruits and vegetables, the body digests and assimilates juices within ten to fifteen minutes of drinking them. Your body makes maximum use of juices to nourish and regenerate your cells, tissues, glands, and organs.

The Healthy Green

It isn't just the mythical Popeye who can benefit from eating spinach. Consider the following:

- If you are feeling "plugged up," instead of turning to expensive over-the-counter remedies for constipation, combine carrot and spinach juice. The same combination serves as a remedy for arthritis, bronchitis, and liver problems. A mixture of spinach and carrot juice will also address liver problems as well as gallstones. Spinach juice is good for ulcers too.

- One of the ways to address the problems of menopause nutritionally is to boost your daily intake of vegetables (including salads). In particular, choose dark leafy vegetables such as spinach, kale, collard greens, broccoli, and cabbage, as well as yams, peppers, and tomatoes.

- Eating folate-rich leafy vegetables such as spinach can safeguard against depression and improve cognitive functioning.

- After a stroke or mini-stroke, one recommended step is to eat foods high in B vitamins and calcium. Examples are dark leafy greens such as spinach and kale, sea vegetables (seaweed), almonds, beans, and whole grains (if no allergy).

Specific juice recipes can target specific conditions. For example, carrots and yams can help improve resistance to allergies. While carrot juice is fine by itself, you can enhance its flavor by adding such combinations as spinach, beets, and cucumbers. Another tasty, superfood drink combination is spinach, kale, celery, and apple, along with either water or coconut water for added flavor.

When it comes to spinach, organic varieties are infinitely better than canned or conventionally grown spinach. Some people argue that it is too costly to buy organic. In reality it is more costly *not to* eat organic. Consider the lower nutritional value of most foods and the sicknesses, diseases, and health care costs that stem from eating them. In the long run spending the extra money is worth it. Organic foods are not sprayed with pesticides or other chemicals and contain lower quantities of toxic trace minerals. Various studies have shown that organic foods contain much more iron, potassium, magnesium, and calcium.

Chapter 9

BERRIES ARE BERRY BERRY GOOD

SCIENTISTS HAVE FOUND that berries have some of the highest antioxidant levels around, making them the most powerful (and delicious) disease-fighting foods available. The color pigments in berries are what give them these powerful antioxidants. Blue, purple, and red pigments have been associated with a lower risk of certain cancers, urinary tract infections, poor memory function, and the effects of aging. Consuming dietary fiber, which is found only in berries and other plant foods, also contributes to these health benefits. You should include different types of berries in your diet, such as strawberries, blueberries, raspberries, blackberries, and cranberries (and no matter what flavor, skip the juice).

Despite their tiny size, berries are powerful sources of phytochemicals—chemicals found in plants that have a variety of beneficial health effects. One phytochemical in particular is ellagic acid, which is believed to help prevent cellular changes that can lead to cancer. The good news is that *all* berries contain some ellagic acid, with strawberries and raspberries ranking among the top sources. Berries and the ellagic acid they contain may help fight cancer on several fronts, according to Gary Stoner, PhD, professor and cancer researcher at Ohio State University in Columbus, who has worked on a number of studies involving blackberries. Dr. Stoner comments: "The National Cancer Institute recommends that every American eat at least four to six helpings of fruit and vegetables each day. We suggest that one of these helpings be berries of some sort."[1]

A University of Georgia lab study found that phenolic

compounds extracted from blueberries could limit colon cancer's ability to multiply and could also trigger renegade cells to die. Thus, their findings suggest that blueberry intake may reduce colon cancer. Blueberries also appear to ward off deadly cancers, while protecting cells against damage caused by diabetes. Additional research suggests that consuming wild blueberries may help protect the brain against cell death due to ischemic stroke, which occurs when the brain is deprived of oxygen and can produce lasting damage to the nervous system.[2]

HEART HEALTHY

Blueberries are an outstanding food when it comes to heart health and lowering blood pressure. When it comes to harnessing the power of antioxidants, in comparison with other fruits and vegetables, blueberries rank number one. Antioxidants help neutralize the damaging effects of free radicals that can lead to numerous diseases, including heart disease, cancer, and Alzheimer's. Specific to the heart, the antioxidants in blueberries work to help reduce your cholesterol, decreasing your risk for heart attack and stroke. Blueberries, as well as strawberries, raspberries, black raspberries, cranberries, blackberries, and other berries have some of the highest antioxidant levels of any fruits.

While berries are typically only available during certain seasons, the most potent form of berries is freeze-dried, which should be available all year round and are great to sprinkle on salads, cereal, or in yogurt. Frozen berries are also a good alternative in smoothies or mixed with fresh yogurt as a cold dessert to replace ice cream. It's best to choose organic berries since berries are prone to contain pesticide residues.

Berry Nutrition

Here are some health tips involving berries:

- To help diffuse stress and its effects, choose blackberries, as well as such foods as fish, beans, broccoli, bananas, and almonds.
- Before hunger pangs or cravings strike, stock up on low-glycemic snacks such as strawberries, grapes, apples, and carrots to keep your blood sugar on an even keel.
- To get inflammation-fighting antioxidants, eat a wide variety of fruits and vegetables, especially blueberries and kiwi fruit.

Another healthy aspect of berries is their flavonoid content; blackberries in particular are among the highest-rated foods containing this class of substances. Other fruits and vegetables are rich in flavonoids, which are chemicals that have attracted considerable attention because of their effects on the cardiovascular system and cardiovascular risk factors. While most fruits and vegetables should be part of a heart-healthy diet, those with high concentrations of flavonol are particularly beneficial. In the Iowa Women's Health Study, investigators followed nearly thirty-five thousand women for sixteen years and found a lower risk of death from heart disease among females with a higher consumption of flavonoid-rich foods.[3]

The Power of Goji Berries

Goji berries are the highest antioxidant energy food on the planet. Why? Because they grow in the highest altitudes on the earth—places like Tibet—and are able to withstand harsh climates where almost nothing else grows. They contain at least eighteen amino acids and are a complex protein, as well as an excellent source of minerals. Along with other raw, high-protein foods such as spirulina, chlorella, and cacao, goji berries also contain tryptophan, which can boost your mood and mental outlook. Among their many benefits, goji berries:

+ Contain 500 times more vitamin C by weight than oranges
+ Have vitamin E, which is nearly unheard of in fruits
+ Have more beta-carotene than carrots
+ Contain B vitamins
+ Help increase testosterone and libido
+ Contain nineteen amino acids, which include eight essential amino acids
+ Contain twenty-one trace minerals, which include zinc, calcium, and selenium
+ Contain beta-sitosterol, which aids in lowering cholesterol and improves sexual health
+ Have antibacterial and antifungal properties
+ Have essential fatty acids, such as omega-6

OTHER BENEFITS

Berries have other benefits, starting with quercetin; leading sources include blueberries, blackberries, cranberries, elderberries, mulberries, and raspberries. Quercetin has such features as helping support the immune system, helping clear excess congestion, and fighting mild allergy problems. It is also used in some weight-control programs. Like other flavonoids, quercetin is an antioxidant that travels throughout the body, removing harmful free radicals. Studies have shown that quercetin may also be a potential solution to cardiovascular disease.

Finally, berries can nourish your brain by increasing levels of GABA and magnesium. Your brain is an extraordinary creation. It houses and expresses your personality, information, past memories, and future desires. It coordinates your consciousness and unconsciousness, and it gives your life impetus and purpose. Using your brain, you can read this book and then go to the kitchen to prepare your next meal.

Recipe: Very Berry Sundae

8 oz. raspberries

12 oz. blueberries

2 Tbsp. fresh orange juice

1 Tbsp. honey

1 tsp. vanilla extract

1/4 tsp. almond extract

1 pint fat-free vanilla frozen yogurt

Place half of the raspberries in a medium glass bowl. Mash lightly with a fork. Add the blueberries, orange juice, honey, vanilla and almond extracts, as well as the remaining raspberries. Stir well to mix. Cover and let stand for at least thirty minutes to allow the flavors to blend.

One of the substances your brain needs is GABA (gamma-aminobutyric acid), a naturally occurring amino acid. It is the main inhibitory neurotransmitter that restores your brain and regulates anxiety, moods, muscle spasms, depression, and chronic stress. For its proper metabolism, other nutrients work along with GABA, in particular, magnesium. Since GABA actually fills the GABA receptor sites in the brain, while mood-altering drugs merely attach to the receptors, proponents believe that by restoring the brain chemistry with GABA and other amino acids, the brain becomes balanced so that sensory reception is sharp, clear, and intact.

Trauma and stress deplete GABA. Emotions such as grief, anger, fear, and anxiety, as well as physical pain, all play a big part in this depletion. When your GABA supply has been depleted, your entire body will tell you. Your eyes will dilate, vision blur, mouth dry, heart race, lungs constrict, and stomach contract. Your adrenal glands will pump out adrenaline, leaving you weak. If left unresolved, you may develop chronic pains, insomnia, panic attacks, headaches, and emotional discomfort.

Another substance with a link to the brain is magnesium. This vital mineral enhances the action and effect of amino acids. The symptoms of magnesium deficiency are the same as those that occur with anxiety, stress, and emotional depletion. They include depression, fatigue, irregular heartbeat, irritable bowel syndrome and spastic symptoms, headaches, noise sensitivity, fibromyalgia, low blood sugar, dizziness, constipation, asthma, and chronic pain.

One of the leading foods to turn around a depletion of magnesium is blackberries. Among others that should be part of your daily diet are almonds, broccoli, green beans, bananas, black-eyed peas, dates, and tuna. Note that even if you eat foods rich in magnesium, you may require a magnesium supplement. Chronic stress makes your blood pressure increase, which causes blood cells to release magnesium into your blood plasma, after which it is excreted in urine.

Chapter 10

APPLES, THE WONDER FRUIT

W**HEN JOHN CHAPMAN**, aka "Johnny Appleseed," wandered around the eastern states and the Midwest during the 1800s to plant apple seeds and establish apple orchards, he did not realize that his efforts would later help significantly improve Americans' health. Since Johnny's days research has shown that eating apples can reduce the risk of heart disease, lower the risk of lung cancer, lower your risk of asthma, and improve lung function.

Apples are high in antioxidants, which have been linked to better heart health. In addition to being a delicious and flexible ingredient, in laboratory studies apples have also been linked to a reduced risk of heart damage. Eating apples and apple products have been linked to providing protection from cellular damage that otherwise could have led to an increased risk of heart disease and certain cancers. An apple or two a day may indeed keep the doctor away. Consider these apple nutrition facts:

- Apples are a natural source of health-promoting phytonutrients, a plant-based antioxidant that promotes bone health.

- Apples contain natural fruit sugars, mostly in the form of fructose, and because of an apple's high-fiber content, the fruit's natural sugars are slowly released into the bloodstream, helping maintain steady blood sugar levels.

- Apples are an excellent source of fiber, containing both soluble and insoluble fiber.

+ Not only are apples fat free, saturated fat free, sodium free, and cholesterol free, they can help lower cholesterol and blood pressure while stabilizing blood sugar.

There are many other health benefits that scientists believe are linked to eating apples and apple products, from fighting Alzheimer's disease and breast cancer to furthering weight loss. Speaking of weight loss, the insoluble fiber found mostly in the skin—the kind we call "roughage"—has long been recommended to prevent constipation. In addition, insoluble fiber is very filling, which is why the apple is a wonderful weight-control food for people who want to lose weight without feeling hungry.

Rapid Immune Fix

Not only can an apple a day keep the doctor away, it can also serve as a rapid fix for your immune system. If struggling with a cold or other virus, try two organic apples (or four organic pears). Apples and pears contain pectin, which help remove toxins, aid bowel movements, drain the lymphatic system, and alleviate swelling in a sore throat and tonsils.

Concerning lung health, a study in the Netherlands found that those who ate more apples and pears had better lung function and less chronic obstructive pulmonary disease. Apples are high in quercetin, an exceptional antioxidant that helps prevent harmful oxygen molecules from damaging individual cells. Consequently apples may also help ward off lung cancer. Finnish researchers found that men who consumed more quercetin were 60 percent less likely to have lung cancer than men with lower quercetin intake.[1]

The Wonder Fruit

Apples can rightfully be termed a "wonder fruit," since they do several things for your health simultaneously. In addition to the benefits listed earlier, apples also combat intestinal infections, inflammation, diarrhea, and an overly acidic stomach. More than half of your immune system is associated with your gastrointestinal tract; apples are excellent for good intestinal health. In addition, apples help the body detoxify and fight viral infections.

While it may sound like an exaggeration to brag so much about apples, if you don't believe it, incorporate one or two organic apples into your daily diet. You will start feeling healthier and more energetic. As this superfood helps fill you up and reduce your appetite, it helps cleanse the liver, gallbladder, and colon. In addition, a tablespoon of raw organic apple cider vinegar a day will help release fat cells, improve digestion, and speed up metabolism.

When you eat them, don't throw out the seeds, the skin, or the core. Did you ever see a horse spit out any part of an apple? There's a reason for the old saying: "He's as healthy as a horse." Horses eat the whole apple and so should you. While you may have heard that apple seeds are toxic, this is not a concern. Although they do contain trace amounts of cyanide, your normal, healthy cells contain an enzyme that renders this cyanide inactive. Interestingly, cancer cells do not contain this important enzyme, so chewing apple seeds can actually help your body kill cancer cells while not harming normal cells.

Another reason to make apples and other fresh fruits and vegetables the cornerstone of your daily diet is the hazards inherent in modern food production. For example, 60 percent of the antibiotics used in the United States are given to animals. In addition to the glut of these substances given to animals, the growth hormones they receive also pass along through the meat you consume. The danger of this? Consuming too many antibiotics means you kill good bacteria as well as bad bacteria in your body. You desperately need that good bacteria at work inside you. You can replenish it by eating apples, as well as figs, pineapples, prunes, yogurt, and cabbage.

ATTACKING FREE RADICALS

The cells of your body are composed of molecules. Molecules consist of one or more atoms, with each proton nucleus being orbited by a number of electrons. Atoms are always seeking to achieve a state of maximum stability by gaining or losing electrons or by sharing electrons with other atoms. When weakened atoms split, they create odd, unpaired electrons, and free radicals are formed. Unstable free radicals try to capture their needed electrons from other compounds to gain stability. They usually attack the nearest stable molecule to "rob" it of an electron, which means that the second molecule now becomes a free radical. This process keeps happening until something stops it, and much damage can be done to cells in the process.

Free radicals arise during normal body metabolic processes, but environmental factors such as tobacco smoke, herbicides, radiation, and pollution can hasten their formation. Naturally, free radical damage becomes more noticeable as a person ages. The only way to retard free-radical damage is to provide the body with antioxidants, which are able to "donate" one of their own electrons without becoming unstable free radicals themselves. Vitamins E and C are especially effective in this regard. In essence, they help to prevent cell and tissue damage that could otherwise lead to serious disease and functional difficulties.[2] As your brain "fires" all day and all night, each of your billions of brain cells has more potential than other cells in your body for free radical damage. You don't want the damage to occur at a faster rate than it can be repaired, or diminished brain function will be the result, somewhat like "rusting out."

Eat More Apples

Knowing you should get more fresh fruit into your daily diet is one thing. Making it happen is another. Fast-faced, twenty-first-century schedules make it easy to fall into the junk-food, fast-food, convenience-food trap. Still, you can combat it by keeping fresh fruits and vegetables on hand. Stock up with fresh organic apples, as well as oranges, grapefruit, and bananas, and when in season include blueberries, strawberries, and melons. Slice, rinse, and store it in easily accessible places, such as in a bowl on the dining room table or kitchen counter.

In foods, antioxidants can often be identified by their bright colors, which is why you are often told to choose an array of colors of fresh produce. Those bright red apples, cherries, and tomatoes, orange carrots, yellow corn and mangos, and dark bluish purple blueberries, blackberries, and grapes abound with antioxidants.[3] The antioxidants that are found naturally in many foods, including fruits and vegetables, nuts, grains, and some meats, include: beta-carotene, lutein, lycopene, selenium, vitamin A, vitamin C, and vitamin E.[4]

It's not a simple cause-and-effect equation. The more scientists research antioxidants, the more complex the story becomes. It isn't the case that massive doses of antioxidants will stave off all cancer, Alzheimer's disease, macular degeneration of the eye, or cardiovascular disease. Still, everyone can benefit from a healthy increase in his or her consumption of those bright-colored fresh fruits and vegetables.

What's the moral of the antioxidant story? The older you are, the lower the level of antioxidants in your body, and the more you need that fresh, unpeeled, organically grown apple instead of that piece of apple pie.

Chapter 11

I YAM WHAT I YAM

A PREVIOUS CHAPTER REFERRED to Popeye's love of spinach. Classic cartoon lovers also remember one of this lovable character's favorite refrains: "I yam what I yam, and that's all what I yam." Popeye wasn't referring to sweet potatoes or their oft-misidentified cousin, yams (sweet potatoes are often labeled as yams to distinguish orange from lighter varieties), but whatever name you use, just like spinach, these flowering plants are healthy powerhouses. They can help preserve memory, control diabetes, reduce the risk of heart disease and cancer, and are a good source of fiber.

Nutrition expert Dr. Don Colbert rates them a top anti-inflammatory food. Along with such foods as spinach, onions, chili peppers, and carrots, sweet potatoes fight high blood pressure. They provide vitamin B_5, which works in conjunction with other B vitamins and with the adrenal gland to fight stress.

Women especially should be aware that sweet potatoes and yams are a rich source of DHEA. This important precursor hormone can become estrogen, testosterone, or progesterone as needed in the body. The problem is, the aging process depletes the body's level of DHEA, which hampers anti-aging defenses. By regularly adding sweet potatoes and yams to your diet, you will receive high amounts of DHEA, as well as beta-carotene, vitamin C, protein, and the aforementioned fiber. All work in symphony to keep the body young, vibrant, and full of energy.

The sweet potato is one of the best friends a woman can have during the perimenopausal and menopausal years. Not only is this bright, luscious powerhouse packed with DHEA, but it also contains vitamin A to boost resistance to infections and allergies, and lots of B and C vitamins. Besides their stress-fighting qualities, these vitamins help fight fatigue. Many studies have shown that a woman can cut her risk for stroke by eating a sweet potato daily.

Since sweet potatoes are a good source of fiber, which helps lower blood sugar levels, they are a wise choice for those with diabetes. Because sweet potatoes are high in complex carbohydrates, they can help people control their weight to help keep diabetes under control. In addition, because sweet potatoes contain the B vitamins folate and B_6, they may give the brain a boost in performing its functions, which sometimes diminish with age.

ANTIOXIDANT STRENGTH

Sweet potatoes contain antioxidants, key tools in the fight against disease. Oxidative damage and the resultant inflammatory changes are now known to lie at the root of most common chronic conditions, such as cardiovascular disease and cancer, in humans.[1] As Popeye might say, "Antioxidants to the rescue!" Antioxidants are a specific group of vitamins, minerals, or other substances that neutralize free radicals in your body, preventing damage to your cells. After they neutralize these free radicals, they become inactive and are eliminated. However, this process means that you continually need to supply your body with antioxidant protection through diet, supplements, or both.

All experts agree that eating whole foods in their natural state, complete with naturally occurring antioxidants, is the best way to go. You should make every effort to eat fresh, healthy food. Still, in this fast-paced society, many people need to resort to supplements to insure they get adequate amounts.

Recipe: Sweet Sesame Potatoes
----

2 pounds sweet potatoes

2 tsp. sesame seeds

1 bunch scallions, chopped

1 clove garlic, minced

1 Tbsp. olive oil

1 Tbsp. Bragg Liquid Aminos

1 Tbsp. packed light brown sugar

1 tsp. dark sesame oil

Scrub the sweet potatoes and pat dry with paper towels. With a fork, pierce each potato in three or four places. Place the potatoes, in spoke fashion and with the thinner ends pointing toward the center, on a paper towel in a microwave oven. Microwave on high power for five minutes. Turn the potatoes. Microwave for five to nine minutes more, or until the potatoes can be easily pierced with the tip of a sharp knife but are still firm. Set aside until cool enough to handle. Peel, then cut into thick slices.

Place the sesame seeds in a large nonstick skillet. Stir over medium heat for thirty seconds or until golden. Stir in the scallions, olive oil, and garlic. Cook for thirty seconds longer or until fragrant. Add the Bragg Liquid Aminos, brown sugar, and dark sesame oil. Cook until the sugar melts, about ten seconds. Add the sweet potatoes to the pan, and toss to coat. Cook for one minute to heat through.

Makes six servings.

Because of their ability to prevent many of the diseases associated with aging, three major antioxidants—beta-carotene and vitamins C and E—should be part of your arsenal of life extenders.

These antioxidants offer a three-point attack in preventing oxidative damage. Beta-carotene quenches single oxygen molecules. Vitamin C protects tissues and blood components. Vitamin E protects cell membranes.

Vitamin E is an antioxidant derived from plants. It is a family of nutrients that include tocopherol and tocotrienols, each with their own subfamilies of alpha, beta, gamma, and delta substances. Vitamin C and beta-carotene also fight free radicals and offer protection against heart disease, cataracts, and certain cancers, including skin cancer. Sweet potatoes (and mangoes) are rich sources of all three.

Junk-Food Junkie

Sweet potatoes, yams, and other vegetables don't rank high on the list of the standard American diet's favorite foods—especially compared to sugar-, fat-, and salt-laden fast food, junk food, and ice cream sundaes. Yet it is these superfoods that ought to come first. Calling sugar "poison" may be overkill, but realistically its overconsumption feeds obesity and other diseases, some of which can be fatal.

To explain: as a whole, cancers feed on sugar. So when you choose to eat sugar, you are giving cancer its favorite food. Cancer cells have metabolisms as much as eight times higher than those of normal cells. So the quick burst of hyper-energy provided by high levels of glucose in your bloodstream create a fertile environment for cancers to develop, grow, and spread. When you consider that high sugar levels impede immune system functions and fan the flames of inflammation, sugar becomes a double ally of cancer. Anyone fighting cancer at any stage should reduce sugar intake.

In addition they should limit high-glycemic foods that can feed cancer. As mentioned in chapters 5 and 8, high-glycemic foods are those that raise blood sugar rapidly. The faster a food is converted to sugar, the more rapidly the blood sugar rises and the higher its glycemic index. The glycemic index (GI) gives an indication of the rate at which different carbs and foods break down to release sugar in the bloodstream. Because these foods cause the blood sugar to rise more slowly, insulin levels do not rise significantly, and the blood sugar levels are stabilized for a longer period of time. One of the most important factors that determine a food's glycemic index value is simply how much the food has been processed.

JUDGE FOOD BY COLOR

The University of Sydney manages a web site at www.glycemicindex .com that shows the ratings of various foods. However, if you don't have a way to easily identify a glycemic index number, here's a rule of thumb: judge by color. White foods (white bread, white sugar, white rice, baked potatoes, and white pastas) tend to be higher than colorful fruits and vegetables, such as sweet potatoes, beans, peas, lentils, and Ezekiel 4:9 bread. The index rating of white potatoes is twice that of sweet potatoes.

According to a recent study, there is evidence that cancer cells also need glutamine, an amino acid, to utilize glucose, and that in the absence of glutamine, glucose will go unused.[2] This research may lead to possibilities for new glutamine-blocking drugs for cancer treatment. However, normal and cancer cells both need glutamine and glucose to function, so as a normal dietary concern for someone without cancer, you are better off decreasing your sugar intake by avoiding high-glycemic foods and sugar than you are worrying about your glutamine levels.

Sweet but Healthy Treat

When buying sweet potatoes, always choose those with the most intense, lush orange color. The richer the color, the

greater the jolt of beta-carotene. Store your "sweeties" at
room temperature to lengthen their shelf life and make sure
not to get them wet, as they will spoil. Wash when ready to
cook them. Once baked, sweet potatoes will keep in your refrigerator for seven to ten days. To prepare for baking, simply
scrub them, dry them, and pierce the skins in several places
with a fork. Place them on a baking sheet because they will drip
juices during the baking process. Bake at 350 degrees for one
hour. For an added treat, sprinkle with cinnamon and brown
sugar and a little butter.

In this category, sodas of all kinds are big violators, even if they
are not sweetened with high-fructose corn syrup. Artificial sweeteners appear to be just as bad as sugars, if not worse. A recent study
estimated that individuals who consume two or more soft drinks a
week have an 87 percent higher risk of pancreatic cancer than those
who don't. Further research into this is needed, however, as drinking
soft drinks is somewhat difficult to separate from other harmful ele-
ments such as smoking, caloric intake, being overweight, and having
type 2 diabetes, since many who drink a lot of soft drinks also par-
ticipate in one or more of these activities as well.[3]

Chapter 12

THE PERFECT POMEGRANATE

THE AMAZING POMEGRANATE represents longevity and immortality in many ancient cultures. Originating in the Persian region known today as Iran, it is one of the oldest known fruits and revered as a symbol of health and fertility in many cultures. Ironically you can't eat its tough outer layer, only the seeds and juice inside. In the case of the pomegranate, digging out the edible parts is indeed like finding buried treasure. It is a nutrient-dense food source and rich in healthy phytochemical compounds.

Aside from its romantic links with the past, today's research shows that pomegranates can help prevent the most common health problems associated with aging, particularly heart disease. Among the heart system's components this amazing fruit addresses is atherosclerosis. It also can improve blood flow and LDL oxidation, and prevent high blood pressure. Laboratory research suggests that it may be effective in such conditions as diabetes, neurological health, infections, and osteoarthritis.

The versatile pomegranate has long been used in folk medicine around the world to treat cuts, sore throats, diarrhea, gum disease, and infections. The aforementioned Greek physician Hippocrates used this fruit for treating fevers. Today it is widely recognized for its antioxidant properties too. Studies show that the pomegranate has more antioxidant power than any of the foods typically recommended as antioxidants, including blueberries, cranberries, red wine, and green tea. It is also more powerful acting than the common antioxidants vitamins A, C, and E. The pomegranate's antioxidant properties are attributed to its high content of soluble polyphenols,

including a tannin called punicalagin. Punicalagins help lower cholesterol and blood pressure and speed up the pace at which blockages melt away. They are the major component responsible for the
antioxidant and health benefits of pomegranate juice.[1]

Helping Your Heart

As mentioned above, the pomegranate is an amazing food when
it comes to helping protect the heart. Its unique properties allow
it to help protect the inner lining of the arteries from damage.
Most of the studies on the pomegranate have focused on its effect
on heart disease. Clinical studies in humans have focused on the
pomegranate's ability to prevent and treat atherosclerosis, diabetes,
osteoarthritis, and cancer. A few studies have also documented the
pomegranate's antibacterial and antiviral effects.

Still, the question remains: Can pomegranates reverse heart disease? According to recent studies, they can. The majority of the
studies on health benefits of pomegranates have explored their
ability to stop and even reverse the buildup of harmful plaque in
blood-carrying arteries. These studies show that pomegranates offer
significant health benefits for people at risk for heart disease. It has
been suggested that pomegranates combat atherosclerosis by stimulating paraoxonase (PON) enzyme activity and HDL-associated
protein. Animal studies show that polyphenols inhibit LDL oxidation and reduce atherosclerosis, thus reducing the risk for cardiovascular problems such as heart attack and stroke.

In addition to its cardiovascular protection, pomegranates
offer help for osteoarthritis by inhibiting cartilage breakdown.[2]
Researchers have also identified two anti-dementia components in
pomegranates: ellagic acid and punicalagin. Both of these components seem to inhibit a serine protease associated with dementia.[3]
Adding other benefits such as improved immune functioning,

neurological health, and protection against cancer and osteoarthritis show the power of the perfect pomegranate.

CANCER FIGHTER

In addition to its anti-inflammatory properties and the way it increases antioxidants in the blood, studies continue to reinforce that pomegranate is a leading cancer-fighter that inhibits hormone-driven cancers. The reason? It is chock full of ellagitannins, which appear to interfere with the hormonal cycles that promote breast and prostate cancers. As it is digested, pomegranate also releases ellagic acid, a compound that promotes the cancer-fighting attributes of this and other berries.

Research is still being done on this wonder fruit, but with pomegranates' ability to fight other illnesses as well, such as arthritis and heart disease, it is worth considering adding a daily glass (2 to 4 ounces) of pomegranate juice to your normal breakfast routine. A study conducted by UCLA researchers found that drinking 8 ounces of pomegranate juice a day decreased prostate cancer significantly. One research study suggested that drinking 50 milliliters (about 1.7 ounces) of pomegranate juice daily for up to a year can lower systolic blood pressure—the top number—readings by 5 to 21 percent. However, drinking pomegranate juice doesn't seem to affect diastolic pressure (the lower number).[4]

Preliminary laboratory research and clinical trials showed that juice of the pomegranate may be effective in reducing heart disease risk factors, including LDL oxidation, macrophage oxidative status, and foam cell formation.[5] In mice, "oxidation of LDL by peritoneal macrophages was reduced by up to 90 percent after pomegranate juice consumption."[6]

Pomegranate also contains a high amount of antioxidants called polyphenols, to which most of the fruit's benefits are attributed. One of the ways pomegranate might lower blood pressure is by inhibiting angiotensin-converting enzyme activity, or ACE, according to a study conducted by researchers at the Rappaport Family Institute for Research in the Medical Sciences in Israel. According to a study reported in a past issue of *Atherosclerosis*, researchers observed that patients with hypertension taking 50 milliliters of pomegranate juice daily for two weeks experienced decreases in ACE activity and reductions in systolic blood pressure.[7]

The Healthy Fruit

The toxic state of the American diet contributes significantly to the higher heart disease rates Americans have in comparison to other countries. What you eat matters. When it comes to heart health (as well as lowering blood pressure), the pomegranate fruit is one of the best things to work into your diet, whether in food or liquid form. It can help prevent and reverse heart disease and dementia, as well as inhibit cartilage breakdown associated with osteoarthritis.

POMEGRANATE'S DIETARY CONTRIBUTION

Numerous dietary issues are behind the Western world's problems with disease, which is why eating superfoods such as pomegranate is so vital to good health. English experts such as J. Yudkin from London, in 1972 and later in 1974, and T. L. Cleave from Bristol reported a high incidence of cancer in peoples from the modern world because of diets rich in fats and refined foods, resulting in constipation. Later T. D. Wilkins and A. S. Hackman published similar findings with respect to Americans.[8] Their feces contained elevated quantities of nitrogen, fat, cholesterol, biliary acids, and a high concentration of carcinogenic metabolites, which are chemical wastes produced as our body metabolizes the adulterated food.

Dr. Adlercreutz, in his article "Diet, Mammary Cancer and Metabolism of the Sex Hormone," underlines the fact that Western women enjoy unrestrained consumption of animal proteins and fats, along with refined carbohydrates. This low-fiber diet increases their risk of colon cancer and substantially increases the production of estrogens. This excessive endogenous estrogen—which normally should be eliminated through the stool—is trapped in the colon by constipation and is easily reabsorbed into the bloodstream. In contrast, Asian women who eat high-fiber, unprocessed foods avoid this deadly cycle. Their hormones tend to be much more stable because of their superior diet and good detoxification. It is now commonly accepted that high-fiber diets increase expectancy for good health.

However, although many estrogen and estrogenic chemicals are harmful, take note that some boost health. The pomegranate and such vegetables as soybeans and broccoli offer phytohormones or phytoestrogens, which protect the body from carcinogenic mutations. Typically, diets that contain good amounts of these and other phytoestrogen-rich foods help fight against disease. Chinese and Japanese women eat foods rich in good estrogen, such as tofu, soy, and miso. They seldom develop cancer, and curiously, they rarely suffer osteoporosis or any of the diseases related to low estrogen production after menopause.

Chapter 13

OATMEAL: BREAKFAST
OF CHAMPIONS

WHEN IT COMES to starting your day with a healthy breakfast, one of the leading options is oatmeal. Just like apples, a bowl of this heart-healthy superfood can also keep the doctor away. For nutrition this whole grain ranks up there with such other meal or snack choices as black beans, kidney beans, citrus fruits, or flaxseed. Oatmeal is a low-calorie, low-fat, high-protein, high-fiber substance that can help slow weight gain by making you feel fuller and less likely to reach for that sugary mid-morning snack. Its soluble fiber can help lower your "bad" LDL cholesterol, prevent hardening of the arteries, and boost your immune system while protecting against heart disease. If that weren't enough, it can reduce the risk of developing diabetes by helping stabilize blood sugar. Plus, it fits the menus of those who must avoid gluten.

Oatmeal can help reduce the development of breast cancer and high blood pressure too and is full of healthy antioxidants and vitamins. Biotin, which is found in B complex vitamins, is a nutrient that forms the basis of skin, nail, and hair cells. Without enough biotin, your skin will lack radiance. One way to get adequate biotin is by eating foods such as oatmeal and bananas (which make a great topping for oatmeal). You probably never imagined that a morning bowl of oatmeal had the potential to transform your skin and help it shimmer with a healthy glow as it retains moisture, stays smooth, and looks younger.

It is a versatile entrée too. You can top your oatmeal with any number of tasty options. Besides bananas you can use blueberries, strawberries, peaches, pears, apples, figs, pineapples, walnuts, and almonds, as well as such spices as cinnamon or nutmeg. Or use oats and fruit to create a breakfast smoothie. A word about the instant varieties: while appealing because of speed and convenience, many of these selections are high in sugar, which helps negate some of oatmeal's health benefits. In this case, slow is better. It will take longer to prepare steel-cut oatmeal, but it will be time well spent. If you choose instant, look for high-fiber varieties.

BOOSTING SEROTONIN

Oatmeal is a natural way to increase your levels of serotonin. In the central nervous system serotonin plays an important role in the regulation of body temperature, mood, sleep, vomiting, sexuality, and appetite. Low levels of serotonin have been associated with several disorders. The most notable include clinical depression, migraine headaches, irritable bowel syndrome, tinnitus, fibromyalgia, bipolar disorder, and anxiety disorders. Lack of serotonin can make you feel irritable, depressed, and unhappy.

Not only can oatmeal boost serotonin, at the end of a long day it can help you fall asleep by serving as a healthy late-night snack without the drawback of unnatural side effects. However, this doesn't mean that oatmeal is a "sure fire" cure to resolving a serotonin shortage. Since lack of sleep is often associated with low serotonin levels, one of the fastest ways to increase serotonin is to get more sleep. When you sleep peacefully and long enough (at least seven hours), you wake up feeling refreshed. Many negative emotions often diminish with a good night's sleep. During deep sleep serotonin levels increase, helping to replenish and renew various parts of the body. Have you ever felt totally hopeless and frustrated—and then took a nap or woke up the next day after a long sleep, and the

issue that seemed like a mountain had turned into a molehill? This
is what higher serotonin levels and sleep can do.

Also, the creative side of your brain is activated when you rest
and sleep more. When you are overworked and don't get adequate
sleep, this shuts down your creativity, awareness, joy, and peace of
mind, which affects your personality. Lack of sleep also increases
phobias, fears, and nightmares. Lack of sleep is a major age accel-
erator. It can weaken the immune system and cause bone loss, skin
dehydration, poor circulation, decline in memory and mental awareness, depression, and other complications.

In his book *Younger You* Dr. Eric Braverman—an expert on
brain chemistry—says that it takes at least seven hours of daily
sleep to boost serotonin levels.[1] Less than forty-nine hours a week
will accelerate the aging process.[2] Some basic things to help you
sleep are avoiding caffeine (not just coffee; countless drinks and
other substances contain it), especially in the evening, and avoiding
electrical input at night, whether through a TV, computer, video
games, or smartphone.

INSOMNIA AND YOUR DIET

Sleep is a supreme tonic. Those who sleep better and know how
to rest or meditate can tap into creativity, new ideas, and a spiritual state much faster than those who try to get by with little rest.
Basically a good night's sleep is like pushing "reset" on your computer when it goes haywire. It is important that you take steps to
sleep deeply and restoratively. If you have trouble getting to sleep
at night or trouble staying asleep all night long, you have insomnia.

A 24/7 Food

Oatmeal is a great idea throughout the day. For starters, it makes a healthy breakfast, thanks to its fiber content. One cup contains 4 grams of fiber, which will help start you on the way to the desired daily average of at least 25 grams. Fiber in that amount or more promotes:

- Better blood sugar control.
- Improved heart disease risk.
- A lower appetite due to feeling full.
- Reduced constipation.
- Reduced risk of colon cancer, irritable bowel syndrome, and diverticulitis.

When you come to the end of the day, oatmeal is still a good idea. Some oatmeal with warm milk can help calm your body down naturally, without the unwholesome side effects of prescription sleep aids.

Insomnia robs your brain of the essential downtime it needs to keep your body's systems running smoothly. A well-rested brain is a healthy brain, and sleep is a supreme tonic. Therefore, it is important that you get deep and restorative sleep every night. Lack of sleep robs your body of the essential downtime it needs to rebuild vital organs and recharge your nervous system. People who return from a restful vacation will say they feel rejuvenated. Friends and coworkers will usually comment on how rested and relaxed they appear. Good, sound, adequate amounts of sleep were probably part of their good vacation. Just think: if it is so evident on the outside, imagine what has taken place inside the person's body, mind, and spirit.

If you have insomnia, it is vital to determine and change the cause of it. It's not going to be enough to pop a pill at bedtime. While prescription sleep aids are popular, they impair calcium absorption, are habit forming, and may paralyze the part of your brain that controls dreaming. As a result, sleeping pills can often impair your clarity of thought and leave you feeling less than rested.

When you are working on reestablishing a healthy sleep pattern, take a hard look at your diet. Are you consuming caffeinated items such as coffee, tea, sodas, or chocolate? Are you consuming them in the evening? Caffeine is a stimulant, and it will keep you awake. What else are you consuming in the evening? It has been said that sleep doesn't interfere with digestion—but digestion does interfere with sleep!

If you are hungry in the late evening, choose a food that will promote relaxation. As mentioned earlier, a small bowl of oatmeal is a good choice, along with such things as a banana, plain yogurt, a small serving of lean turkey or tuna, or a few whole-grain crackers. If you aren't concerned about too much liquid late at night, a cup of chamomile tea right before bed is also good. Chamomile is considered to be a nerve restorative that helps quiet anxiety and stress, probably because it is high in magnesium, calcium, potassium, and B vitamins.

Chapter 14

PROTEIN POWER OF TURKEY

GIVEN ITS HALLOWED place at millions of tables at Thanksgiving and Christmas, turkey includes pleasant connotations associated with good food, friends, and family. However, turkey should grace your menu beyond special holidays as a good source of low-calorie, low-fat protein. Protein equals energy. Consuming quality protein at meals helps give you the energy you need and will provide your body with slow-burning fuel throughout the day.

Lean turkey is a leading source of good-quality protein. Among others are lean chicken, fish, beans, nuts, and seeds. Protein sources contain tyrosine, the amino acid that helps produce neurotransmitters that keep you mentally alert. Tyrosine helps to build the body's natural supply of adrenaline and thyroid hormones. Proteins and amino acids are the body's building blocks. They are used to repair and maintain tissues such as muscles, connective tissue, skin, and bone matrix. If you do not have adequate protein, you will not be able to adequately maintain these tissues, as well as enzymes, hormones, and the immune system. As a result, you will age faster and eventually develop disease.

In 2002 the National Institutes of Health advised that protein should make up 15 to 35 percent of daily consumption of energy or total calories. Anything more than 35 percent as protein is too much; one doctor advises that a maximum of 10 percent come from animal protein. This typically translates into 3 ounces of animal protein once or twice a day for women and 3 to 6 ounces of animal protein once or twice a day for men. Additionally, men should limit red meat to 12 ounces a week, which is where lean meats such as turkey can serve more than one purpose.

Nor is animal protein with every meal necessary. For example, beans and a small amount of brown rice (the size of a tennis ball) is a complete protein. This helps to create the correct fuel mixture that keeps your appetite controlled, your energy up, and your blood sugar and insulin levels in check. Free-range or organic lean turkey is one of the best animal proteins you can choose, along with things such as organic free-range chicken; wild-caught, low-mercury fish; and organic low-fat dairy. These are free of hormones and antibiotics that can be harmful to the body.

Two cautions with turkey:

+ Remember that too much protein can have a negative impact. Studies have shown that men with diets high in red meat have an increased risk of prostate cancer—and it is typically a more aggressive form. Also, frying or grilling meat (including turkey), chicken, or fish so it is charred or well done is associated with an increased risk of cancer.

+ While generally healthy, this refers to the white meat. Three ounces of roasted, white-meat turkey contain just 54 calories and has 2 micrograms of health-building chromium. It is also a top anti-inflammatory food. However, you should avoid or limit dark meat, which has more fat, and avoid the skin.

HEALTHY DIETS

Dr. Janet Maccaro recommends turkey as part of a healthy, high-fiber diet that can help control your weight. She says a high-fiber diet is necessary because fiber improves the excretion of fat, improves glucose tolerance, and gives you a feeling of fullness and satisfaction.

In addition to turkey, she suggests chicken, tuna, white fish, fresh fruits and vegetables, lentils, beans, and whole-grain breads. She also suggests adding healthy fats to your diet, such as olive oil, safflower oil, and flax oil.

Conversely, Maccaro advises avoiding sugars and snack foods that contain salt and fat, such as potato chips, ice cream, candy, cookies, cake, high-sugar breakfast cereals, and sodas. Other prohibitions: high-fat cheeses, sour cream, whole milk, butter, mayonnaise, fried foods, peanut butter (unless natural), rich salad dressings, and alcoholic beverages—the latter because they are so high in calories.

Her guidelines for balanced weight loss:

1. Eat three meals and two snacks daily to keep blood sugar levels stable.

2. Eat protein at each meal in the form of lean meat, eggs, soy, and tofu.

3. Eat plenty of fruits and vegetables at each meal: five servings daily (½ cup is one serving).

4. Watch portion sizes. A meal-sized serving of protein is about the size of your fist.

5. Consume refined grains with caution.

6. Drink plenty of water daily.

To show the importance of "quality" protein to your diet, one 6-ounce portion of lean chicken provides your body with 85 grams of protein. Fish is a concentrated source of protein too, providing about 41.2 grams per serving. An 8-ounce container of yogurt (depending on the type) will give you 8 to 13 grams of protein, and a half a cup of tofu, about 10.1 grams.[1] Ideally, adults need 7 to 9 grams of protein for every 20 pounds of their body weight.[2] So if you weigh 150 pounds, you need to eat about 50 grams of protein daily to stay healthy. (A lack of protein means your body can start to break down its own tissues.)

Her final suggestion when it comes to diet is eating a number of smaller or modest meals interspersed with nourishing snacks, instead of the typical American "three square meals a day" or skipping meals.

HEALTH BOOSTER

Health expert Dr. Don Colbert also recommends organic or free-range poultry (white breast meat with no skin) two to three times a week as part of a healthy diet that can combat cancer. His poultry recommendation compares to his advice that you limit organic or free-range lean red meat to three times a month. Instead of featuring red meat as a main course, he believes in using small amounts as an additive to spice up soup or pasta.

"Why am I so particular about the types of meat I recommend?" he asks. "Cancer patients need adequate protein intake but not the toxic processed meats, such as bologna, bacon, sausage, or excessive amounts of red meat or pork. Instead, they need plant protein, such as beans, lentils, peas, legumes, nuts, seeds; healthy grains such as sprouted breads, wild or brown rice, millet, and others; organic eggs (two to three eggs with only one yolk), chicken and turkey without the skin; wild salmon, sardines, and tongol tuna; and small amounts of organic, grass-feed beef."

Sleep-Promoting Snack

Everybody thinks of turkey as a source of tryptophan when they think of a natural sleep inducer. However, tryptophan will work better when your stomach is *not* overstuffed as it might be on a holiday, and it works better in combination with some complex carbohydrates. If you're about to go to bed, your body does not appreciate a protein overload. So if you are looking for the best mid-evening, sleep-promoting snack, take *just one* slice of lean turkey and enjoy it on a slice of whole grain bread.

Not only should you choose wisely when it comes to turkey and other forms of protein, it also helps to eat protein first instead of the bad habit some have of consuming dessert first to make sure they have room for it. Eating protein first helps boost glucagon levels. Glucagon is a hormone that works totally opposite than insulin works. Insulin is a fat-storing hormone, whereas glucagon is a fat-releasing hormone. In other words, glucagon will enable the body to release stored body fat from the fatty tissues and will permit muscle tissues to burn fat as the preferred fuel source instead of blood sugar.

How do you release this powerful substance into your body? The release of glucagon is stimulated by eating a correct amount of protein in a meal along with the proper balance of fats and carbohydrates. When the insulin levels are high in the body, the level of glucagon is low. When glucagon is high, then insulin is low. When you eat a lot of sugar and starch, you raise your insulin levels and lower your glucagon, thus preventing fat from being released to be used as fuel. By stabilizing blood sugar and lowering insulin levels, you can keep glucagon levels elevated, enabling your body to burn off the extra fat.

Chapter 15

THE STRENGTH OF SALMON

S ALMON. NOT EVERYONE likes it because some varieties have a rather strong "fishy" taste. This may call for using a different method of cooking or additives such as a glaze to enhance the flavor, but the effort will be worth it. Salmon is a great source of protein and one of the healthiest fish you can eat. Wild salmon is one of several cold-water varieties (along with cod, sardines, and tongol tuna) that are a natural source of vitamin D for bone strength and fats that are beneficial for heart health.

Oily fish such as salmon and mackerel should be a regular feature of your diet. Oily fish are rich in omega-3 essential fatty acids, which provide a huge range of health benefits, including helping reduce your level of triglycerides. Triglycerides are "bad fats" in the blood that increase your risk of heart disease. Omega 3s help keep the blood thin, reducing the risk of clots from sticking to arterial walls—a primary cause of fatal heart attacks. They also help reduce the occurrence of dangerous heart arrhythmias and decrease inflammation in the body. The American Heart Association (AHA) recommends eating 3 to 6 ounces of oily fish at least twice per week.

Your body needs fatty acids to survive and is able to make all but two of them—linoleic acid and linolenic acid. These two fatty acids must be supplied by our diets and are therefore considered essential fatty acids (EFAs). EFAs help protect blood vessels from excessive plaque buildup, reduce inflammation throughout the body by stimulating the production of leukotrienes (which are natural compounds that inhibit inflammation), prevent high blood pressure, and help contribute to respiratory health.

There is mounting evidence that suggests that supplementation with omega-3 fatty acids, as well as increased consumption of fruits and vegetables, significantly decreases the chances of developing dementia or Alzheimer's disease.[1] The goal here is to consume all of the omega-3 oils that you can because of their far-reaching health benefits. The AHA published a study of 11,323 heart attack survivors showing that those who took 1,000 mg. of fish oil supplements every day were 45 percent less likely to be dead at the end of 3.5 years.[2]

If you prefer to get most of your omega 3s from food, remember that when it comes to fish, make sure it is wild and low in mercury; steer away from farmed fish of any kind. Fish with the least amounts of mercury include salmon (fresh or canned) as well as anchovies, catfish, crab, flounder, haddock (Atlantic), herring, sardines, shrimp, sole, tilapia, trout (freshwater), and whitefish.[3]

HEART-HEALTHY ESKIMOS

The people of Greenland's Inuit tribes illustrate the benefits of eating oily fish such as salmon. More than fifty years ago reports surfaced about the low prevalence of heart disease among these indigenous Eskimos. Today we know the reason for this stemmed from their diet, composed primarily of whale and seal. These meats are rich in omega-3 (n-3) fatty acids. Along with a "heart-healthy" lipid profile, studies of the Inuits show they have reduced platelet activity and a lower incidence of immune and inflammatory diseases.

Polyunsaturated fats have a chemical structure made up of more than one double bond ("poly" meaning "many"). These fats are named according to the number of double bonds, configuration, and position on the fat chain. The n-6 and n-3 fatty acids—linoleic acid and alpha-linolenic acid (ALA), respectively—are essential nutrients for mammals. Our bodies lack the enzymes needed to synthesize them.

Walnuts and plant oils are good sources for both, especially soybean, flaxseed, linseed, and canola oils. Humans are able to convert linoleic acid and ALA ingested from plants into eicosapentaenoic acid (EPA) and docosahexaenoic acid (DHA), the n-3 fatty acids most relevant in protecting the heart. However, this conversion from plant oils and nuts is fairly limited. Consequently, the main dietary source of n-3 fatty acid is not from plants but fish, especially oily varieties such as salmon, mackerel, trout, herring, and sardines.

Salmon: Good Fat

All fats are not our enemy. We need to learn to choose the good fats and avoid or limit the bad, inflammatory fats. Adequate fat intake helps you maintain your protein so that your body doesn't burn protein as fuel. Fats are also the building blocks for cell membranes. A list of healthy fats starts with fatty fish such as wild salmon. Some other healthy fats are found in sardines, tongol tuna, anchovies, almonds, almond butter, macadamia nuts, avocados, guacamole, pecans, and cashews.

Not only does salmon contain good fats, it can also help you arm yourself against the effects of long-term stress. Flounder, seafood, brown rice, almonds, garlic, lentils, sunflower seeds, bran, and avocados are also good stress-fighters.

Subsequent studies of other populations showed the same protective effects from diets rich in omega oils. There is a clear, well-documented inverse association between fish consumption and heart disease. As the amount of fish in the diet *increases*, the risk of cardiovascular disease *decreases*. Fish oil has several beneficial effects on the heart. It improves the lipid profile by lowering triglycerides and increasing HDL cholesterol. It lowers the heart rate and blood pressure and helps blood vessels and the heart muscle to relax.

PROMOTING HEALTHY TEETH

In addition to promoting heart health, salmon is part of a natural foods diet that can promote healthier teeth and gums. One cornerstone of a tooth-promoting regimen is a diet centered on raw grass-fed dairy products, including raw organic eggs, raw milk, raw cheese, raw cream, and butter is paramount for healthy teeth.[4]

Some of you may be totally opposed to the idea of any dairy or fish—especially if you follow a vegan diet. However, with dairy the problem is not milk itself but all the processing it goes through. Raw and organic milk and raw cheese contain live enzymes and other raw nutrients needed to reverse the decay process in teeth and help to remineralize the enamel, but pasteurization destroys these enzymes. This diminishes the vitamin content and destroys the B_{12} and B_6 vitamins. With the milk's proteins altered and its beneficial bacteria killed, it is no longer a natural food. Instead it has turned into a highly processed junk food that many rightfully claim causes allergies, heart disease, colic in infants, growth problems among children, osteoporosis, arthritis, and even cancer—and increases tooth decay.

If you are a vegan, you can still opt out of eating meat, but increasing raw dairy intake will make a huge difference! In addition to raw dairy, other foods that are good for dental health are organs of sea animals and uncooked or slightly cooked wild salmon and sashimi, and rare or seared tuna. Bone broths, such as fish stew broth, are very mineralizing for teeth. Bone broths make a good stock that you can use as a base for a soup or to flavor other dishes.

DEALING WITH STRESS

Feeling stressed out in today's hyperspeed-paced world? While salmon won't cure everything rushing at you, it can be part of a balanced eating-and-exercise plan that will relieve stress.

Good nutrition is the first key. Start by eliminating caffeine, refined sugars, and carbohydrates from your diet. Then eat at least four servings of fruit and vegetables and three servings of whole grains daily, as well as healthy protein from sources such as salmon and flounder. This will keep you energized and less apt to fall prone to "stress" eating. Your diet should also contain seafood, brown rice, almonds, garlic, lentils, sunflower seeds, bran, brewer's yeast, avocados, and green superfoods such as Kyo-Green (available at your local health food store), which contain protein and all the B vitamins.

Exercise is a huge stress reliever. It helps bring down your high levels of cortisol while increasing endorphins and serotonin, which will inhibit the stress response. Exercising for thirty minutes a day five times a week, along with strength training twice a week, will do wonders for your outlook. So will breaks throughout the workday and taking your dog for a walk or playing with your children.

The other key to dealing with stress is addressing the mental component. Learning to relax is one of the most crucial components of reducing the effects of stress. When you are highly stressed, your adrenal glands are in trouble; this is why you must address the lifestyle habits that are destroying them. Don't forget the value of adequate sleep. Trying to "run on empty" in hopes of getting more done will only deplete and destroy your body—and it's tough to accomplish anything from six feet under.

Chapter 16

CITRUS: NATURAL SUNSHINE

CITRUS FRUITS ARE famous for their vitamin C, a valuable antioxidant linked to all kinds of wonderful benefits. Among them are increasing the absorption of iron in food, helping neutralize free radicals and possibly protecting against heart disease by boosting blood flow through coronary arteries. These fruits are also among the best sources of flavones, as well as fiber, folic acid, and potassium. They also contain limonoids, which have been shown to have powerful anticancer characteristics. Since these are not found in any other fruit except citrus, this makes their cancer-fighting potential unique.

When you mention citrus fruits, most people think primarily of oranges, lemons, limes, and grapefruits. However, as mentioned in chapter 1 on tomatoes, items such as pineapples, tomatoes, kumquats, mandarin oranges, and tangerines are also good choices. Studies from around the world have time and again linked the consumption of citrus fruits (not juices) with a decreased risk of developing different cancers, especially those of the digestive tract: esophageal, mouth, larynx, pharynx, and stomach. Results varied, but most showed a decrease of 40 to 50 percent.[1]

One of the most powerful flavonoids found in citrus fruit is quercetin. Research over the years has shown quercetin to stimulate the system's ability to tear apart tumors, salvage free radicals, inhibit the division of cancer cells, prohibit cell mutation, lessen angiogenesis, and encourage apoptosis. Citrus pectin, a polysaccharide found in the cell wall of citrus fruit, has been shown to decrease metastases in animal studies of prostate cancer and melanoma.[2]

Again, while further study is needed to fathom the full depth of anticancer potency in these fruits, there is certainly enough evidence that citrus should be an important component of the fruits and vegetables that you eat on a daily basis for their health benefits. The juice of lemons or limes squeezed into a glass of water make a delicious beverage; these fruits are also very alkanizing for the tissues.

Not only does citrus contain plenty of vitamin C, it also has lesser amounts of vitamin E. Both can provide your face a natural lift without undergoing a face-lift. How? They improve skin health by countering the damaging effects of sun exposure. Simply leaving the house without sunscreen can cause skin to age prematurely and become dry and wrinkled. Even worse, prolonged sun exposure can lead to skin cancer. Yet your skin needs vitamins C and E desperately on a daily basis. This is where citrus fruits such as oranges, grapefruits, and lemons can provide your skin a robust vitamin C treatment from the inside out.

PESTICIDE-FREE ENVIRONMENT

Citrus can play a valuable role in achieving a pesticide-free diet and environment, as difficult as that goal can be. In today's world we are bombarded with toxins that can over time damage our health—especially the pesticides used in agriculture to protect crops from insect damage and infestation. It is imperative that you become proactive when it comes to limiting exposure to these toxins on a daily basis because they have a cumulative effect that can contribute to diseases such as cancer.

Produce with the lowest amounts of pesticide residue are hard-skinned fruits such as citrus, pineapples, and melons, and such vegetables as squash, corn, and avocados. Foods with the highest residue levels include some items that can be peeled, such as zucchini, cucumbers, peaches, and plums. Given our pesticide-laden environment, grapes, cherries, celery, strawberries, and tomatoes are best eaten when organic.

Concern about pesticides should extend beyond the dinner table to the rest of your home and yard. The pesticide sprays used to kill ants, roaches, and more are made up of chemicals that can shorten your life span. Researchers have found that children living in households that use pesticides have a much higher risk of developing childhood leukemia. You should choose today's new "chemical-free" pest controllers that are available at most health food stores.

There's more. Chlordane, a pesticide composed of over fifty different chemicals and mimics estrogen, was banned in the United States over fifty years ago. But it has continued to be manufactured in the States and shipped to Mexico, where it is sprayed on food crops exported back to the States. According to the Agency for Toxic Substances and Disease Registry, almost every human on earth has chlordane in their fat. There is no way to get it out of the body. Losing weight only concentrates the chemical in the remaining fat.

Reducing Pesticide Exposure

As good as citrus fruits are for your health, the modern use of pesticides calls for care in selection of both fruits and vegetables. Here are some tips:

- Choose hard-skinned fruits—citrus, pineapples, melons—and vegetables, such as squash, corn, and avocados.
- Peel soft-skinned fruits and vegetables, or eat organic fruits and vegetables.
- Wash the foods you are going to eat.
- Do not plant near a house foundation that could have been treated with chlordane.
- Cook with curcumin, also known as turmeric.

Besides being sprayed on America's corn, millions of tons of chlordane were put into the ground around house foundations to kill termites before it was banned. The half-life of chlordane in soil is twenty-two years. This means that it will not degrade for at least forty years.[3] The good news is that curcumin (an herb from India also called turmeric) has been shown to have the ability to block many dangerous chemicals, including chlordane.[4]

ADDRESSING MENOPAUSAL MOODS

Women who are in the perimenopausal or menopausal stage of life should pay attention to the benefits of citrus. Boosting daily intake of fruits such as oranges and lemons, as well as melons, bananas, and dried fruit (apricots, figs) will increase your potassium levels. Potassium-rich foods help balance sodium and water retention. Among other steps that can help address menopause are eating plenty of fiber; one way is to add regular helpings of beans and lentils to meals. Also, stop frying foods; broil or bake them instead. Boost your daily intake of vegetables, including salads.

You should also get rid of white bread and products made from white flour while choosing whole-grain breads, oats, rye, and wheat germ. Eat fewer regular white potatoes and more sweet potatoes, and eliminate white rice (except basmati) and switch to long-grain brown rice. Replace processed cooking oils with unprocessed oils and use extra-virgin olive oil, canola, and flaxseed oil. Make oily fish such as salmon and mackerel part of your diet. Drink more mineral/ bottled water, less caffeine, and little to no alcohol. Consume high-calorie junk foods only occasionally, as a treat.

To help you during menopause, try adding seaweed to your diet. Choose nori, wakame, kombu, and arame, which contain natural hormones and plant chemicals.

MIGRAINE RESTRICTION

Even though citrus is one of twenty-one superfoods we recommend, there is a caution involved with their consumption (which is one reason we suggest consulting a physician or dietician about any eating plan). Though ordinarily healthy, citrus, bananas, avocados, and chocolate are some foods that you may need to limit or avoid if you are suffering from migraines.

Because the brain is the control center of your body, any disease or unhealthy influence that it suffers can have far-reaching effects on the rest of your body, not to mention your ability to reason clearly and to remember things. One of the most common brain-related complaints is the common headache; the more serious are known as migraines. As most people know, a migraine can arise from various causes, including anxiety and stress, lack of food or sleep, exposure to bright light, or, in women, hormonal changes. The pain is often centered in a particular location, and it seems to pulse or throb.

Sufferers become sensitive to light and sound, and they may become nauseated to the point of vomiting. Some people can tell when a migraine is about to start because they see flashing lights or have other visual disturbances.[5] Nutritionally, what can you do about migraine headaches is to avoid potential headache-trigger foods.[6]

In addition to avoiding citrus and chocolate, you need to be wary of cheese, anything prepared with monosodium glutamate (MSG), foods containing the amino acid tyramine (found in red wine, aged cheese, smoked fish, chicken livers, figs, and some beans), nuts or peanut butter, onions, dairy products, meats containing nitrates (bacon, hot dogs, salami, cured meats), and fermented or pickled foods. By trial and error and guidance from a doctor or health specialist, you can tailor your diet to your own situation.

Chapter 17

FAT-BURNING GREEN TEA

ADVERTISING OF FRAUDULENT diet products and fat-burning agents is so common the Federal Trade Commission (FTC) warns on its website that anything promising weight loss without sacrifice or effort is bogus. Here's good news about green tea, though: While drinking it isn't a sure-fire, single-method way to shed weight, it can help burn off fat naturally. Green tea has thermogenic properties, a term that describes the body's natural means of raising its temperature to burn calories. It is the process of triggering the body to burn white body fat, the kind often accumulated by the aging process. Thermogenic agents are fat burners that help to increase the rate of white-body-fat breakdown.

This is why green tea and green tea extract make good weight-loss supplements. It is one of the two best teas—the other being yerba mate—for providing natural energy and speeding up metabolism. Green tea has two key ingredients: a catechin called epigallocatechin gallate (EGCG) and caffeine. Both lead to the release of more epinephrine, which then increases the metabolic rate. Ultimately green tea promotes fat oxidation, which is fat burning. It also increases the rate at which you burn calories over a twenty-four-hour period. An effective daily dose of EGCG is 90 milligrams or more, which can be consumed by drinking three or four cups of green tea a day.

While the FTC's statement illustrates the fact there are many questionable weight-loss products on the market, there are a variety of safe and effective over-the-counter supplements for weight loss. Some people may find that incorporating a combination of these into their eating and activity plan works. However, rather than relying on just supplements or swallowing the kind of phony claims warned against by the Federal Trade Commission, why not incorporate natural substances such as green tea?

The truth is that there is no shortcut to losing weight and keeping it off. A new lifestyle that includes good nutrition, exercise, supplementation, and constant diligence is the best way to overcome obesity. While vitamins and supplements can help, eating superfoods such as green tea and others reviewed in this book can fuel a new lifestyle characterized by health and vitality.

CANCER FIGHTER

More than a good fat burner, green tea also helps fight cancer. The polyphenols in tea, especially the catechins, are powerful antioxidants that help ward off cancer as well as diabetes. Green tea has a four-thousand-year history of treating a wide variety of ailments. Chinese people have been touting the benefits of green tea since before their first dynasty. In the United States back in 1944 an article published by the National Cancer Institute showed that a regular diet that included green tea could reduce the risks of esophageal cancer by as much as 60 percent. The study also found that certain compounds found in green tea tended to inhibit the growth of cancer cells.

Also, laboratory research has shown time and again that green tea catechins, including EGCG, reduce the growth of various kinds of cancer cells. A landmark study presented in 2005 by researchers from two Italian universities recently demonstrated that green tea catechins were 90 percent effective in keeping men with premalignant lesions in the prostate from developing prostate cancer.[1] In fact, more than 135 different studies have supported the claim that ingesting certain levels of green tea helps to fight cancer.

EGCG is readily absorbed into the body and has been shown

to promote cancer cell apoptosis and prevent angiogenesis, and it has important antioxidant properties. It has also been shown with epicatechin-3 gallate (ECG)—another component of green tea—to indirectly lower the synthesis of dihydrotestosterone, which has been identified as an accomplice in contributing to prostate cancer and enlargement. Researchers at the University of Rochester in New York also recently announced that EGCG targets heat shock protein 90, a protein present in cancer cells more than normal cells.[2] This protein makes the cells resistant to chemotherapy and radiation therapy, so EGCG shows promise in thwarting the growth and survival of cancer cells already under treatment.

Green tea catechins also appear to have chemopreventive effects on colon, rectal, lung, stomach, and kidney cancers, as well as prostate cancer. Research has long shown that cultures that drink a good deal of green tea (such as several in Asia) have lower incidences of various kinds of cancer. In fact, despite Japan's high smoking rate, its rates of lung cancer remain consistently lower than Western countries.[3]

Green Tea Boost

As mentioned elsewhere in this chapter, green tea is high in an antioxidant known as epigallocatechin gallate, or EGCG. Clinical tests show that EGCG:

- Inhibits the growth of new cancer cells but kills some existing cancer cells without harming normal cells.

- Inhibits the unnatural formation of blood clots, which have been known to cause thrombosis, one of the leading causes of heart attacks and stroke.

- Reduces total cholesterol levels and increases the ratio of HDL (good cholesterol) to LDL (bad cholesterol).

In addition, green tea is a good anti-aging prescription since it contains a rich source of antioxidants and substances that assist detoxification. Plus, it can help keep your bones healthy. This is especially important to women, who tend to lose 1 to 3 percent of their bone mass yearly during the first five to ten years after entering menopause.

HEART HEALTHY

The free-radical inhibiting property of tea is more potent than that of vitamin E and is a proven preventative and treatment for atherosclerosis, otherwise known as hardening of the arteries. A large, population-based study in Japan found that the higher green tea consumption, the lower the risk of death from cardiovascular disease.[4] While all of tea's heart protective effects are not clear, it does lower total and LDL cholesterol levels, which is one possible mechanism. In animal studies tea showed reduced absorption of cholesterol from the intestines, reduced the amount of cholesterol produced by the liver, and increased the amount of cholesterol excreted in the feces.

Green teas represent a rich source of flavonoids, while black tea contains theaflavin, a product derived from the fermentation of green tea to form black tea. Both have favorable effects on cholesterol levels. In one study involving 240 men and women with high cholesterol—and who were already on a diet low in saturated fat—participants who took theaflavin-enriched green tea extract experienced a significant drop in LDL cholesterol levels, compared to those who took a placebo.[5]

While tea should not replace a statin in people with high risk for heart disease, it can be used in addition to one. For men and women at low risk for heart disease, but who have mild to moderately elevated cholesterol, green tea is worth trying in conjunction with diet modification.

GABA Booster

Mentioned previously in chapters on broccoli and berries, GABA is a chemical in the brain that causes you to relax, reduces anxiety and stress, and increases alertness, which is why some call it the "peacemaker" chemical. GABA keeps all the other neurotransmitters and hormones in check. People who are GABA-deficient can become irritable and unfocused, experience chronic anxiety, and have difficulty handling the day-to-day stresses of life. Symptoms can also include headaches, palpitations, heart disorders, low sex drive, and hypertension.

Although there are prescription medications that can help the GABA receptors, unfriendly side effects can often accompany them. So the best, safest way to achieve natural health is with diet, natural supplements, and spices. Citrus fruits are among the foods that increase GABA levels, as well as almonds, bananas, lentils, brown rice, spinach, halibut, and whole grains.

A supplement that helps boost GABA levels is L-theanine, which calms nerves and increases mental clarity. This amino acid is also found in green tea, which makes an excellent way to start the day. So chuck the phony diet products and brew yourself some green tea. Your body will be glad you did!

Chapter 18

FLAX: TINY SEEDS, HUGE PAYOFF

W HILE THE SEEDS of the flax plant only measure a fraction of an inch, don't let their tiny size fool you. Flaxseeds are a source of such minerals as iron, zinc, calcium, and magnesium, as well as vitamin E and folate. They are also one of the best sources of omega-3 fatty acids that are incredibly beneficial for your health. Despite the low-fat craze of recent years, you shouldn't avoid fats entirely. Instead, increase your awareness of bad fats and good fats as part of a search for ways of eating more healthy fats.

Bad fats include trans fats and refined omega-6 fats, such as most commercial oils, salad dressings, gravies, sauces, and deep-fried foods. Fats that are good in moderation but bad in excess are saturated fats and unrefined omega-6 fats, such as cold-pressed vegetable oils. Among good omega-3 fats are flaxseed, salba seed, hemp and chia seed, and oils made from these seeds, fish oils, and monounsaturated fats, such as extra-virgin olive oil, avocados, almonds, and other nuts and seeds.

While eating too much fat can make you obese, avoiding unhealthy fats is different than simply shunning all fats. Fats help absorb important vitamin D and other fat soluble vitamins, including vitamins A, E, and K. Adequate fat intake helps you maintain your protein so that your body doesn't burn protein as fuel. Fats are also the building blocks for cell membranes. Both flaxseed and flaxseed oil contain healthy fats that should be part of your dietary regimen, particularly if you are currently fighting or have any concerns about any genetically linked forms of cancer. Cancer interferes with fat

storage, as these various forms of disease makes the body less efficient in storing fat. This is one of the reasons most patients with
advanced cancers look so thin and emaciated.

This is where flaxseed can be so valuable. It is one of the richest
sources of plant lignans, which act as plant hormones and inhibit
the effects of testosterone and estrogen on hormone-sensitive cancers such as those in the prostate and breasts. These lignans work to
alter estrogen metabolism, block angiogenesis, and encourage apoptosis in these cancers. (One caution here is that flaxseed oil does not
have the high lignan content that flaxseeds do.) In a recent study
of three thousand women, eleven hundred of whom had confirmed
cases of breast cancer, researchers deduced that premenopausal
women with a high lignan intake reduced their risk of cancer by
about 44 percent.[1] One of these flaxseed lignans, enterolactone, was
found in another study to have "a strong protective effect on breast
cancer risk."[2] Another study found that men with the highest levels
of enterolactone were 82 percent less likely to have prostate cancer.[3]

HEART-HEALTHY FOOD

Flaxseeds are more than a good fat. They are a heart-healthy superfood. This is because flaxseeds are a polyunsaturated fat. Such
fats have a chemical structure made up of more than one double
bond ("poly" meaning "many"). These fats are named according to
the number of double bonds, configuration, and position on the fat
chain. The n-6 and n-3 fatty acids—linoleic acid and alpha-linolenic
acid (ALA), respectively—are essential nutrients for mammals. The
human body lacks the enzymes needed to synthesize them. Walnuts
and plant oils are good sources for both, including flaxseed, soybean,
linseed, and canola oils.

Ample Omega 3s

Flaxseed isn't the only way to add healthy omega-3 oils to your diet; you can simply eat more fish for dinner. However, flaxseeds can add variety to your diet. In addition to sprinkling them in soups or salads, the oils of flaxseed, perilla, and fish are ways to get more omega 3s. You can also try sprinkling flaxseeds on oatmeal or into fresh fruit smoothies. Why is it so important to get more omega 3s? Populations that get ample amounts of these essential acids show the lowest rates of cardiovascular disease and the highest percentage of healthy and robust seniors.

As noted in chapter 15, the main dietary source of n-3 fatty acid is not plants but oily fish. However, although fish ranks ahead of flaxseed in heart protection, that doesn't mean you should ignore these powerful little seeds. They can be added to your diet either whole or ground up, although ground flaxseed provides more nutritional benefits because it is easier to digest. As with so many foods, though, moderation is key. Flaxseeds are calorie-dense, so a couple tablespoons per day is sufficient.

Flaxseeds can play a key role in increasing fiber consumption too—something that is a good tool for any eating plan. This means such steps as increasing the fruits and vegetables you eat and replacing breads and cereals made from refined flours with whole-grain breads and cereals. Eating foods such as flaxseeds, chia seeds, hemp seeds, pumpkin seeds, sunflower seeds, old-fashioned steel-cut oatmeal, and sprouted breads such as Ezekiel 4:9 will set you on a road to better health.

DEALING WITH MENOPAUSE

Flaxseed oil is one of the dietary methods available to women dealing with symptoms of perimenopause that normally appear around the age of forty. This oil will help increase intake of essential fatty acids, which will help to reduce pain due to bloating, breast tenderness, endometriosis, and menstrual cramping. Essential fatty acids are also good for skin, hair, and the heart. You can get more of these omega 3s by replacing processed cooking oils with unprocessed oils. Substitute flaxseed, extra-virgin olive, or walnut oils for safflower, sunflower, corn, sesame, and other polyunsaturated vegetable oils.

The perimenopausal stage usually continues until the early fifties, when the menstrual period becomes a thing of the past, signaling the beginning of menopause. During this stage of life, many women experience a decrease or even a cessation in their progesterone production because of irregular ovarian cycling and ovarian aging. At the same time estrogen levels may be excessively or moderately high, causing a troubling, continual state of imbalance.

Women may experience a plethora of symptoms, some for years on end. These may include mood swings, fatigue, breast tenderness, foggy thinking, irritability, headaches, insomnia, decreased sex drive, anxiety, depression, allergy symptoms (including asthma), fat gain (especially around the middle), hair loss, memory loss, water retention, bone loss, slow metabolism, endometrial and breast cancers, and many more. In other words, hormonal imbalance has far-reaching effects on many tissues in the body, including the heart, brain, blood vessels, bones, uterus, and breasts.

The key to smooth perimenopause is bringing the levels of estrogen and progesterone back into balance as well as managing stress. To bring the hormone levels back into balance, doctors prescribe natural progesterone. According to the late pioneer of progesterone therapy, John R. Lee, MD, "One of progesterone's most powerful and important roles in the body is to balance and oppose estrogen."[4] Natural progesterone has been found to be effective in combating perimenopausal anxiety and mood swings. In addition, it plays a very important part in the prevention and reversal of osteo-porosis. Natural progesterone offers a woman all of these benefits without hormone replacement therapy (HRT). The recommended dosage for women in perimenopause is a quarter to a half teaspoon applied to any clean area of skin twice a day (morning and evening). There are natural supplements that you can use to deal with any of the perimenopausal symptoms you are experiencing.

In addition to cooking with flaxseed oil, try the following peri-menopausal marvels in your daily regimen:

+ Quercetin is a potent antioxidant that reduces the inflammation of endometriosis. It also helps reduce estrogen and cholesterol levels while boosting circula-tion and proper digestion.

+ Chaste tree berry promotes progesterone production.

+ Bromelain is a digestive enzyme that reduces pain and inflammation when taken between meals.

+ Vitamin C has additional wide-reaching benefits.

Chapter 19

DARK CHOCOLATE DREAMS

ADMIT IT: WHEN you saw "chocolate" in the table of contents, you couldn't resist turning first to this chapter. Chocolate is derived from cacao beans that were revered by the Aztecs, who believed that eating chocolate would confer wisdom and vitality. While chocolate as a health food may seem like a stretch, it's true. However, only with the precaution to choose dark chocolate over milk chocolate, and then only in small quantities. How small? A small square of a chocolate bar or a bite the size of one Hershey's kiss. An ounce and a half of dark chocolate a day should give you the maximum benefit from this "luxury food" without tipping the balance in the wrong direction because of its high sugar and fat content.

When it comes to chocolate, the darker the better. Why? Because the darker the chocolate, the higher the cacao concentration. Though cacao beans are roughly 50 to 57 percent fat, the good fats (oleic acid, a monounsaturated fat also found in olive oil) outweigh the bad in dark chocolate, so it is neutral in its effect on blood cholesterol. The same is not true of milk chocolate. Dark chocolate has a relatively low glycemic index rating, but the level of a particular selection depends on its sugar content. Because of these attributes, if eaten in moderation, dark chocolate can enhance healthy desserts—such as berries—or serve as part of a high-energy snack. It can help in other ways, such as by providing magnesium, which relaxes tense muscles.

The reason dark chocolate could be worth its calories is that it is full of polyphenols. Fifty grams of dark chocolate has more polyphenols than a cup of green tea and about twice that of a glass of red wine. Chocolate also contains proanthocyanidins. Research has found that the proanthocyanidins can slow the progress of certain cancers (particularly lung cancer) and inhibit angiogenesis. Though more research is needed to confirm these findings, there is growing evidence that these proanthocyanidins interfere with several events in the formation and progression of cancers, thus tripping it up and slowing it down enough for a healthy immune system to deal with easily.

A POTENT SUBSTANCE

A potent antioxidant, dark chocolate contains plant phenols—cocoa phenols, to be exact—that are known to lower blood pressure.[1] A report published by Cochrane Collaborations that analyzed twenty studies found that people who ate a bit of dark chocolate or cocoa daily experienced a slight reduction in blood pressure. The researchers discovered that flavonol-rich chocolate or cocoa powder reduced blood pressure on average by 2–3 mmHg, a measurement related to pressure readings.

Researchers also discovered that when people consume antioxidants in chocolate called flavonols, the body produces a substance called nitric oxide. The chemical "relaxes" blood vessel walls, allowing blood to pass through with less obstruction.[2] Some doctors recommend some chocolates with high cocoa content (at least 70 percent) to patients with high blood pressure who have been instructed to lower their salt and carbohydrate intake.

While watching your consumption is a necessary part of enjoying chocolate, it literally can make you feel good. Endorphin secretion may be triggered by the consumption of certain foods, such as chocolate and chili peppers. Indeed, the characteristic increase in bodily endorphin levels caused by chocolate could explain why we often turn to it as a comfort food in times of stress. Chocolate is by far the most popular endorphin-producing food on the earth. It contains more than three hundred different compounds, including anandamide, a chemical that mimics marijuana's soothing effects on the brain. It also contains chemical compounds such as flavonoids (also found in wine) that have antioxidant properties and reduce serum cholesterol.

Although the combined psychochemical effects of these compounds on the central nervous system are poorly understood, the production of endorphins is believed to contribute to the renowned "inner glow" experienced by dedicated chocolate lovers. What's more, for those who grow ecstatic at the mere mention of the word, there is other good news. Cocoa exhibits effects similar to tea on the cholesterol profile, with a reduction in LDL cholesterol and elevation of the good HDL. In addition, cocoa contains a blood-pressure-lowering effect and may decrease insulin resistance.

However, keep in mind that there is a big difference between natural cocoa and milk chocolate—which is why we specify dark. Milk chocolate is a combination of cocoa, sugar, milk, and other ingredients that can contribute to weight gain, which "presumably" may increase cardiovascular risk. However, this can't be stated with certainty because at least one meta-analysis of several observational studies found a reduced rate of cardiac and metabolic diseases (including stroke) in people who had a higher consumption of chocolate.[3]

OTHER CHOCOLATE CAVEATS

Just as we warned against consuming too much dark chocolate, there are a few other caveats with this sugary treat, starting with women struggling with premenstrual syndrome, or PMS. Diet is a key to managing these problems, which includes avoiding chocolate and refined sugars. Even though the amount of caffeine in chocolate is small, if you have PMS you should avoid caffeine and chocolate to ease water retentiveness.

You should also limit animal products in your diet (buy organic if you eat any meat) and choose low-fat foods and seafood. Eat plenty of cruciferous vegetables (broccoli, cauliflower) and dark, leafy greens to reduce estrogen buildup, and brown rice for its B vitamins. Buy organic milk, milk products, and canned foods, and eliminate dairy products during premenstrual days. Use whole grains, and keep your diet low in sugar and salt.

To keep your bowel function optimal, add fiber to your diet and drink plenty of water. To help control premenstrual cravings for sweets, increased appetite, headaches, and fatigue, consider the following supplements:

+ Balanced B-complex vitamin: 50–100 mg of each B vitamin
+ Chromium picolinate: 200 mcg daily (400 mcg if over 150 pounds)
+ Calcium: 800–1,200 mg daily
+ Magnesium: 400–800 mg daily

Aside from PMS, if you are having difficulty sleeping or establishing a healthy sleep pattern, consider eliminating chocolate from your diet. Chocolate and other caffeinated items—coffee, tea, and sodas—serve as stimulants that keep you awake. They activate your nervous system, other major body systems, and cause your level of adrenaline to rise. This causes an increase in heart rate, breathing rate, digestion speed (more stomach acids), and urinary output (because of its diuretic effect).

Not only should you avoid chocolate at bedtime, but also any meals that include ham, bacon, sauerkraut, sausage, cheese, eggplant, spinach, tomatoes, sugar, or wine. All contain tyramine, which encourages the release of norepinephrine, which is a brain stimulant. Chinese food is another late night no-no if you are sensitive to additives, preservatives, or agents such as MSG, often found in Chinese foods. For some people these substances have a stimulant effect.

GENETIC FACTORS

Family history is another consideration when it comes to chocolate. Does your family history include diabetes? Or do you crave sweets at certain times of the day or when you are under stress? Do you consume ice cream, chocolate, pies, cakes, and candy more than twice a week? Do you crave sodas or other sweetened drinks? Do you feel weak and shaky if your meal is delayed? Do you feel tense, uptight, and nervous at certain times during the day?

Not Always a Treat

While dark chocolate can be good for you, take care in the selection and quantity you consume. For example, those struggling with a sugar addiction or obesity are likely better off skipping chocolate. So are those who have problems with inflammation in their body; among the foods on a list of things to avoid are Hershey Kisses, Twix, Almond Joy, Snickers, and any other kinds of milk chocolate bars. Plus, those who struggle with headaches should avoid chocolate.

If these feelings are familiar to you and your food choices are loaded with sugar, you must focus on eating more fiber and protein foods at each meal and cutting back on simple sugar. Not only should you avoid chocolate, but also such foods as sweet-tasting desserts and snacks, dried fruits, canned fruits packed in sugar syrup, sweetened milk products, and all foods (whether sweet tasting or not) processed with sugar (look for "sugars" on the nutritional label). As a substitute sweetener, you can use honey, rice syrup, or fructose (sugar derived from fruit).

Chapter 20

YOGURT: YOUR GUT
WILL THANK YOU

Y OU ARE NEARING the end of our list of superfoods, which wouldn't be complete without yogurt. This creamy substance can serve as a healthy breakfast, a low-calorie dessert, or a late-night snack that won't keep you awake. Chances are you picked up this book in an effort to learn more about healthy eating, which starts with common sense. For example, it may be popular to chow down on a breakfast of bacon and eggs and pancakes, but it isn't wise. You would be much better off starting the day with low-fat yogurt, a slice of whole-grain toast, and a banana or a handful of almonds. Choosing the right breakfast will enhance your energy and make you less susceptible to reaching for sugary snacks during the day.

However, yogurt demands wise choices. The best ones are Greek yogurt, fat free, and organic without added fruit. If you are not open to fat free, at least choose low-fat yogurt. Frozen yogurt and the endless varieties of fruit-flavored yogurt that are heavily advertising on television and in cyberspace also contain a lot of high-fructose corn syrup. This sweetener is particularly bad for efforts to keep your weight under control.

The careful selection required for yogurt parallels the challenge of changing your daily menu to achieve better health. Shifting eating patterns doesn't mean denying yourself the things you love as much as searching for new alternatives. While greasy burgers and ice cream sundaes are pleasing for a short time, a constant diet of them can prove fatal in the long run. This will require some counter-food-cultural living and different meal preparations. Still, it will be worth the self-control necessary to form new, healthier habits. Yogurts can replace ice cream and cake, fish and salad can replace beef and potatoes, and oranges and apples can be snacks instead of candy bars and chips.

Yogurt is a "live" food. Eating a whole-food, live diet is like a preventative medicine. It promotes health by decreasing fats and sugar intake while increasing fiber and nutrient intake. In addition, it means more satisfaction and less overeating. Also, whole-food diets are low in fat and cholesterol but high in essential nutrients—unlike foods many Americans normally eat that rob the body rather than nourish it. These "robbers" include refined sugars, commercial colas, white flour, and hydrogenated fats such as margarine.

A whole-food diet will allow you to experience optimal and vibrant health. Besides fermented dairy products such as yogurt and kefir, this means such items as various colored vegetables and fruits, grains, raw seeds, nuts, and their butters, beans, fish, and poultry. This kind of diet contains the kinds of foods that are as whole to their original state as possible, and with the least amount of processed, adulterated, fried, or sweetened additives.

Good for Your Gut

There is more to yogurt than its "living" characteristics. Yogurt contains probiotics, which are live microorganisms thought to be healthy for the host organism. Probiotics are commonly consumed as part of fermented foods with specially added active live cultures. Probiotics are beneficial bacteria in your intestinal tract that can improve health by maintaining and boosting the gastrointestinal and immune system functions. In other words, eat yogurt, and your gut will thank you.

Probiotics act with a part of your small intestine called the

Peyer's patches, which directly tell your immune system to be vigilant. Probiotics produce volatile fatty acids that provide metabolic energy. In addition, they help you digest food and amino acids, produce certain vitamins, and, most importantly, make your lower intestine mildly acidic, thus inhibiting the growth of bad bacteria such as E. coli, which has caused serious illnesses in recent years.

Probiotic supplementation is essential in the fight against any fungal infection because of the antifungal properties that these "natural defenders" possess. Everyone has needed an antibiotic at one time or another; yeast infections, gastrointestinal distress, and diarrhea have plagued millions. Antibiotics may help wipe out an infection by killing off bad bacteria. Unfortunately they assault good bacteria as well. That leaves you without the full arsenal of gastrointestinal protection that probiotics supply.

According to the best-selling book *Prescription for Nutritional Healing*, the flora in a healthy colon should consist of at least 85 percent lactobacilli and 15 percent coliform bacteria.[1] The typical colon bacteria count today is the reverse, which for millions has resulted in too much gas, bloating, intestinal and systemic toxicity, constipation, and malabsorption of nutrients, making the colon a perfect breeding ground for the overgrowth of candida.

While probiotics can be taken in a powder, capsule, or liquid form, it is best to obtain them from food sources whenever possible. For optimum probiotic activity, look for yogurts that contain bifidobacterium and/or lactobacilli. In addition to yogurt, some other sources are buttermilk, goat's milk, miso, kimchi, and sauerkraut. If your work or travel schedule limits your options, there are probiotic drink mixes that can be found at health food stores that contain beneficial probiotic organisms.

Path to Total Health

In addition to choosing plain, fat-free, or low-fat yogurt, if you hope to walk the path to total health you should stop eating pasteurized dairy products of any kind. While the raw varieties are fine, pasteurized milk, cheese, and yogurt go through a process that destroys all the enzymes and nutrients, leaving digestive and other complications. When it comes to yogurt, eating non-pasteurized versions allows you to avoid the problems of pasteurization while getting its benefits. Among them are calcium, protein, and magnesium.

You can increase the amount of calcium in your diet by eating yogurt, as well as low-fat cottage cheese, skim milk cheeses, almonds, sunflower seeds, soy, and parsley. Or try taking a calcium-magnesium supplement containing 400 milligrams of calcium and 200 milligrams of magnesium two times a day. However, new studies are finding that consuming over 1,000 milligrams of calcium a day in foods and supplements can increase the risk of heart attack and stroke. So don't overdo it on calcium supplements, and don't consume excessive dairy products.

Yogurt is a good source of protein, which should be part of every meal. Protein will help to give you the energy you need and provide your body with slow- and even-burning fuel throughout the day. As mentioned in chapter 14, an 8-ounce container of yogurt (depending on the type) will give you 8 to 13 grams of protein.

Yogurt is also a good source of potassium. It isn't quite as easy to get adequate amounts of this healthy mineral. In order to switch to a diet higher in potassium, you need to know which foods to choose. Although in recent times lawmakers have considered requiring food manufacturers to include potassium content on food labels, just as sodium is already listed, it has remained optional. Such labeling would allow shoppers to see the amount of each and calculate the ratio in the supermarket. However, until such a change is made, choose good sources. Besides yogurt, an ideal way to get more potassium is selecting foods that don't even need a nutrition label, such as fresh produce and plant-based foods. Foods such as whole grains, legumes, nuts, seeds, fruits, and vegetables all fit the bill.

Probiotic Health

As mentioned in this chapter, raw, low-fat yogurt is a healthy source of probiotics, the "good" bacteria that include numerous benefits. Probiotics can:

- Help manage food allergies
- Strengthen your immunity
- Fortify your intestinal tract

Probiotics should be part of a life-extending regimen. In addition to yogurt, other wonderful sources of probiotics are buttermilk, soy milk, and sauerkraut. You may also take probiotics in a capsule, powdered, or liquid form. Look for lactobacillus and acidophilus at your local health food or the refrigerator section of a supermarket.

Chapter 21

BEANS: TAKE A BOW

BEANS ARE A frequent source of jokes. Renowned cancer physician Francisco Contreras likes to tell one about the former patient who shared a favorite memory about his father. Describing her tugging at his sleeve, he relates how she asked, "You know what I remember about your father? He made me laugh—really laugh." Then she asked the question he had once posed to her: "What do you get when you mix onions and beans?" When Dr. Contreras shrugged, she replied, "Tear gas!" and laughed heartily at the memory.

That may be more amusing than some of the stories you've heard about this "musical fruit," but the health benefits of beans are no laughing matter. Beans are a brain-healthy food and a rich source of fiber, B vitamins, calcium, magnesium, and folic acid. A heart-healthy superfood, they are a great substitute for red meat and other forms of animal protein. The premise of the current high-protein diet craze is that carbohydrates cause weight gain by releasing insulin, which stores fat. High-protein advocates say that, instead of eating carbohydrates, you should eat proteins, which will suppress your appetite and help you lose weight. However, one leading health expert points out that carbohydrates contribute to weight gain *only* when they don't contain fiber and when they are eaten in excess.

The Power of Potassium

Potassium is a mineral that helps to lower blood pressure and keep your body's sodium level down to acceptable levels. This why eating foods high in potassium can help protect against high blood pressure. Beans, especially lima beans and soybeans, are an excellent source of potassium. Look for these other high-potassium foods when you shop:

- Tomatoes
- Prunes
- Avocados
- Bananas
- Peaches
- Cantaloupes

Also, a form of seaweed called dulse is extremely high in potassium, with more than 4,000 milligrams of potassium in just one-sixth of a cup. You can find dulse at health food stores.

In fact, fiber-rich carbohydrates such as beans, whole-grains, and fresh vegetables are the most filling foods with the fewest calories. High-protein diets often restrict the intake of many grains, fruits, and some vegetables, which then limits nutrient intake and can contribute to several diseases. For example, meat protein is high in saturated fat and cholesterol and is therefore strongly linked to cardiovascular disease and cancer.

Keep in mind that a high-protein diet (over 100 grams per day) can also weaken your bones because digesting and eliminating protein's by-products makes the body more acidic. This is especially true for red meat because of its tough, fibrous protein content that requires a lot of digestive acids to break it down. So it is wise to get your daily protein requirement from vegetarian sources such as beans, peas, and soy foods. In addition, you may get your quota from meats that are high in omega-3 fatty acids, such as salmon and tuna.

However, while beans have less fat than meat, that doesn't mean you can eat as much as you want. If weight loss is a primary goal, you should limit yourself to 1 cup per day, and no one should eat more than 4 cups. Also, if you haven't eaten beans regularly, you may need to pick up some Beano, an enzyme that helps digest beans and minimize gas.

A HEALTHY DIET

Beans are an integral element of the previously mentioned Mediterranean diet, a hot topic in the health world. There is strong evidence confirming that adapting this eating style can lower the risk for developing many diseases, particularly heart disease. While more than a dozen nations border the Mediterranean Sea and each has cultural nuances affecting diet, there are still some key similarities to the way people in this region eat. Their diets are quite different from the typical Westerner's.

A Mediterranean diet is generally plant-based, consisting primarily of vegetables, fruits, whole grains, beans, nuts, and seeds. Though not necessarily vegan, it features a limited amount of meat, eggs, and dairy products; the meat tends to be fish and poultry, with little red meat. It is worth noting that in some Mediterranean cultures the proportion of total fat in the diet is relatively high and may exceed the amount of fat in the Western diet. However, the predominant type of fat is monounsaturated, derived from plants (specifically olive oil) rather than saturated animal fat.[1]

This diet derives roughly 30 to 40 percent of its calories from healthy fats (foods such as olive oil, avocados, nuts, and fish) and about 40 to 50 percent from healthy carbohydrates such as beans, fruits, vegetables, peas, lentils, and whole grains. Researchers also surmised that it was not any one component of this diet that makes it preventative, but the overall combination of foods. Another element is their avoidance of foods that are potentially harmful, such as excessive calories from omega-6 oils, butter, sweets, and meats.

Combined with daily exercise, this is a powerful diet for living a longer and healthier life. Another study estimated that up to 25 percent of the incidence of colorectal cancer, about 15 percent of the incidence of breast cancer, and about 10 percent of the incidence of prostate cancer could be prevented if we shifted from a common Western diet to a traditional Mediterranean one.[2]

NEEDED ADJUSTMENTS

Although many health experts believe in the Mediterranean diet as the foundation of meal planning, you may need to make adjustments. For example, although breads and pastas are staples in this region, those seeking to lose weight may want to avoid wheat and corn products, at least until they reach their desired waist measurement. If you are suffering from inflammation-related ailments, such as high blood pressure, colitis, reflux, or prediabetes, you will also need to choose foods that do not create an inflammatory response in your body.

Grazing for Health

While eating often throughout the day may seem like a strange way to lose weight, frequent "grazing" is Dr. Don Colbert's number one dieting rule for the patients he counsels who suffer from obesity and diabetes. Dr. Colbert recommends eating lots of salad and vegetables for small meals, as well as beans, peas, or lentils once or twice a day—a total of 1 to 4 cups.

Another consideration is your digestive system. For some people, specific foods have the same effect as a heavy meal, even when consumed in small to moderate quantities. This means some people need to avoid foods such as beans, cucumbers, and peanuts. They can't sleep well with the discomfort of gas production and internal rumblings. Even if they fall asleep quickly because of the full feeling, the extra work their digestive system does will keep waking them up, causing a light sleep.

Combating Disease

Beans are also an effective tool in fighting cancer and diabetes.

Instead of meat, cancer patients need the kind of protein that beans and other foods—lentils, peas, legumes, nuts, seeds, wild millet, chicken, and wild salmon—offer.

Colorful fruits and vegetables are also good, such as sweet potatoes, peas, lentils, and citrus.

Those struggling with cancer should know that in order not to feed cancer, it's best to avoid refined sugars, refined flours, and artificial sweeteners (especially foods and beverages that contain aspartame, which has its own links to cancer). Dark chocolate, which we mentioned in chapter 19, is better than lighter chocolate.

Beans and foods such as fruit, chickpeas, carrots, squash, oat bran, barley, and rice bran, are all good sources of soluble fiber. Fiber is an essential tool for those who are struggling with diabetes or have concerns about prediabetes, which is a precursor of the disease. Studies conducted by James W. Anderson, MD, of the University of Kentucky, showed that high-fiber diets lowered insulin requirements an average of 38 percent in people with type 1 diabetes and 97 percent in people with type 2 diabetes. This means that almost all of the people suffering from type 2 diabetes who followed Dr. Anderson's high-fiber diet were able to lower or stop taking insulin and other diabetes medications and still maintain a healthy blood sugar level. Additionally these results lasted up to fifteen years.[3]

While high-fiber foods such as beans will help lower blood sugar, this doesn't mean they are the sole way to address diabetes. Type 1 diabetics must avoid sugar altogether while limiting starches and fruit, which can cause blood sugar to spike. They must also avoid fruit juices. Type 2 diabetics may benefit from small amounts of low-glycemic fruit that is high in fiber, such as pears and Granny Smith apples. However, those must be used conservatively. Type 2 diabetics should not drink fruit juice or eat applesauce. The most important dietary advice for any diabetic is to avoid sugar and limit refined starches, including white breads, refined pasta, potatoes, most cereals, white rice, and other highly processed foods.

NOTES

Chapter 1—Terrific Tomatoes

1. E. Giovannucci et al., "A Prospective Study of Tomato Products, Lycopene, and Prostate Cancer Risk," *Journal of the National Cancer Institute* 94, no. 5 (March 6, 2002): 391–398.
2. S. Agarwal and A. V. Rao, "Tomato Lycopene and Its Role in Human Health and Chronic Disease," *Canadian Medical Association Journal* 163, no. 6 (September 19, 2000): 739–744; S. Franceshi et al., "Tomatoes and the Risk of Digestive-Tract Cancers," *International Journal of Cancer* 59 (1994): 181–184.
3. E. Giovannucci, "Tomato-Based Products, Lycopene, and Cancer: Review of the Epidemiologic Literature," *Journal of the National Cancer Institute* 91 (1999): 317–331.
4. Q-Y Lu et al., "Inverse Associations Between Plasma Lycopene and Other Carotenoids and Prostate Cancer," *Cancer Epidemiology, Biomarkers and Prevention* 10, no. 7 (July 2001): 749–756.
5. Richard Béliveau and Denis Gingras, *Foods to Fight Cancer*, 136.
6. *The New York Times*, "Tomatoes Found to Cut Risk of Prostate Cancer," December 7, 1995, http://tinyurl.com/nocam89 (accessed February 24, 2014).
7. Béliveau and Gingras, *Foods to Fight Cancer*, 141.

Chapter 2—Great Grapes

1. Medline Plus, "Antioxidants," U.S. National Library of Medicine and National Institutes of Health, http://www.nlm.nih.gov/medlineplus/antioxidants.html (accessed February 9, 2014).
2. USDA Database for the Flavonoid Content of Selected Foods, Release 3 (2011), US Department of Agriculture, http://tinyurl.com/kftdea7 (accessed February 24, 2014).
3. J. Constant, "Alcohol, Ischemic Heart Disease, and the French Paradox," *Coronary Artery Disease* 8, no. 10 (October 1997): 645–649; J. D. Folts, "Potential Health Benefits From the Flavonoids in Grape Products on Vascular Disease," *Advances in Experimental Medicine and Biology* 505 (2002): 95–111; Luis Bujanda et al., "Effect of

Resveratrol on Alcohol-Induced Mortality and Liver Lesions in Mice," *BMC Gastroenterology* 6 (November 14, 2006): 35.

4. H. Nakagawa et al., "Resveratrol Inhibits Human Breast Cancer Cell Growth and May Mitigate the Effect of Linoleic Acid, a Potent Breast Cancer Cell Stimulator," *Journal of Cancer Research and Clinical Oncolology* 127, no. 4 (April 2001): 258–264.

5. B. D. Gehm et al., "Resveratrol, a Polyphenolic Compound Found in Grapes and Wine, Is an Agonist for the Estrogen Receptor," *Proceedings of the National Academy of Sciences of the United States* 94, no. 25 (December 9, 1997): 14138–14143.

CHAPTER 3—NUTS TO YOU!

1. D. J. Jenkins et al., "Effect of Almonds on Insulin Secretion and Insulin Resistance in Nondiabetic Hyperlipidemic Subjects: A Randomized Controlled Crossover Trial," *Metabolism* 57, no. 7 (July 2008): 882–887.

2. G. E. Fraser et al. "A Possible Protective Effect of Nut Consumption on Risk of Coronary Heart Disease (The Adventist Health Study)," *Archives of Internal Medicine* 152, no. 7 (July 1992): 1416–1424.

3. G. E. Fraser et al., "Association Among Health Habits, Risk Factors, and All-Cause Mortality in a Black California Population," *Epidemiology* 8 no. 2 (March 1997): 168–174.

4. F. B. Hu and M. J. Stamfer, "Nut Consumption and Risk of Coronary Heart Disease: A Review of the Epidemiologic Evidence," *Current Atherosclerosis Reports* 1 no. 3 (November 1999): 204–209; G. E. Fraser and D. J. Shavik, "Ten Years of Life: Is It a Matter of Choice?" *Archives of Internal Medicine* 161 no. 13 (July 9, 2001): 1645–1652.

CHAPTER 4—CELERY: POWERFUL HEALER

1. Anne Hart, "Can Celery Really Lower Your Blood Pressure and Starve Cancer Cells?", Examiner.com, http://tinyurl.com/d2vrlr2 (accessed February 24, 2014).

2. The World's Healthiest Foods, "Celery: What's New and Beneficial About Celery," WHFoods.com, http://tinyurl.com/jhrpd (accessed February 24, 2014).

3. M. A. Gates et al., "Flavonoid Intake and Ovarian Cancer Risk in a Population-Based Case-Control Study," *International Journal of Cancer* 124, no. 8 (April 15, 2009): 1918–1925.

4. Gabriel Cousens, *There Is a Cure for Diabetes* (Berkeley, CA: North Atlantic Books, 2008), 190–200.

5. As referenced in Heather Hudak, "Calm Your Nerves and Love Your Liver With Celery," *Hudak Holistic Health* (blog), July 7, 2010, http://tinyurl.com/o6qb62y (accessed February 24, 2014).

6. FoodReference.com, "Celery Facts and Trivia," http://tinyurl.com/q5c7j52 (accessed February 24, 2014).

7. The World's Healthiest Foods, "Celery: What's New and Beneficial About Celery,"

8. Become Gorgeous, "Health Benefits of Celery Juice," May 5, 2010, http://tinyurl.com/pmmy3v4 (accessed February 24, 2014).

9. Raw Juice Cleansing Recipes, "Health Benefits of Celery Juice," http://tinyurl.com/od4pp6b (accessed February 24, 2014).

Chapter 5—Sprouting Health

1. Johns Hopkins Medicine, "Cancer Protection Compound Abundant in Broccoli Sprouts," September 15, 1997, http://tinyurl.com/b635l6 (accessed February 24, 2014).

2. Gabriel Cousens, "A Healthy Perspective of Sprouts," as quoted in Ellen Schutt, "Proteins and Vitamins and Enzymes, Oh Sprouts!" *Nutraceuticals World*, May 1, 2006, http://tinyurl.com/l7zeghf (accessed February 24, 2014).

3. *USA Weekend*, "Chromium, the Forgotten Fuel," January 12, 1997.

4. Selene Yeager and the editors of *Prevention* magazine, *The Doctors Book of Food Remedies* (New York: Rodale Press, 2007), 222.

5. A. Catharine Ross et al., eds., *Modern Nutrition in Health and Disease Eleventh Edition* (Baltimore, MD: Lippincott Williams & Wilkins; 2012), 159–175.

Chapter 6—Go For Garlic

1. R. McCaleb, "Anticancer Effects of Garlic—More Proof," *Herbal-Gram* 27 (1992): 22–23.

2. S. Foster, "Garlic," Botanical Series 311 (Austin, TX: American Botanical Council, 1991).

3. F. G. McMahon and R. Vargas, "Can Garlic Lower Blood Pressure? A Pilot Study," *Pharmacotherapy* 13, no. 4 (July–August 1993): 406–407, http://tinyurl.com/748qvww (accessed February 24, 2014); WebMD, "Find a Vitamin or Supplement: Garlic," http://tinyurl.com/8654woj (accessed February 10, 2014).

4. G. Li, et al., "Antiproliferative Effects of Garlic Constituents on Cultured Human Breast Cancer Cells," *Oncology Reports* 2 (1995): 787–791.

5. C. Borek, "Antioxidant Health Effects of Aged Garlic Extract," *Journal of Nutrition* 131, no. 3s (March 2001): 1010S–1015S.

Chapter 7—Mighty Mushrooms

1. Sissi Wachtel-Galor et al., eds., *Herbal Medicine: Biomolecular and Clinical Aspects*, 2nd edition (Boca Raton, FL: CRC Press, 2011).

2. Yeager and the editors of *Prevention* magazine, *The Doctors Book of Food Remedies*.

3. K. C. Kim and I. G. Kim, "Ganoderma Lucidum Extracts Protects DNA From Strand Breakage Caused by Hydroxylradical and UV Irradiation," *International Journal of Molecular Medicine* 4, no. 3 (September 1999): 273–277.

Chapter 8—Spinach: Popeye Knew His Stuff

1. S. C. Larsson, E. Giovannucci, and A. Wolk, "A Prospective Study of Dietary Folate Intake and Risk of Colorectal Cancer: Modification by Caffeine Intake and Cigarette Smoking," *Cancer Epidemiology Biomarkers and Prevention* 14, no. 3 (March 2005): 740–743.

2. Inna I. Kruman et al., "Folic Acid Deficiency and Homocysteine Impair DNA Repair in Hippocampal Neurons and Sensitize Them to Amyloid Toxicity in Experimental Models of Alzheimer's Disease," *Journal of Neuroscience* 22, no. 5 (March 1, 2002): 1752–1762.

3. Based on chart at BestDietTips.com, "Glycemic Index Food List (GI)," http://tinyurl.com/d29u6md (accessed February 24, 2014).

Chapter 9—Berries Are Berry Berry Good

1. Holly Wagner, "Black Raspberries Show Multiple Defenses in Thwarting Cancer," *Research News*, Ohio State, October 28, 2001, http://tinyurl.com/5kweht (accessed February 24, 2014).

2. M. I. Sweeney et al., "Feeding Rats Diets Enriched in Lowbush Blueberries for Six Weeks Decreases Ischemia-Induced Brain Damage," *Nutritional Neuroscience* 5, no. 6 (December 2002): 427–431.

3. J. Mink et al., "Flavonoid Intake and Cardiovascular Disease Mortality: A Prospective Study in Postmenopausal Women," *American Journal of Clinical Nutrition* 85, no. 3 (March 2007): 895–909.

CHAPTER 10—APPLES, THE WONDER FRUIT

1. Yeager and the editors of *Prevention* magazine, *The Doctors Book of Food Remedies*, 31.

2. For more information, see "Understanding Free Radicals and Antioxidants" at http://tinyurl.com/8p768 (accessed February 11, 2014).

3. International Food Information Council Foundation, "Functional Foods Fact Sheet: Antioxidants," October 15, 2009, http://tinyurl.com/43q2zun (accessed February 24, 2014).

4. Medline Plus, "Antioxidants," U.S. National Library of Medicine and National Institutes of Health, http://tinyurl.com/cocjgk (accessed February 24, 2014).

CHAPTER 11—I YAM WHAT I YAM

1. J. Guz, T. Dziaman, and A. Szpila, "Do Antioxidant Vitamins Influence Carcinogenesis?" *Postepy Higieny Medycyny Doswiadczalnej* (Warszawa) 61 (2007): 1851–1898.

2. ScienceDaily.com, "Does Sugar Feed Cancer?" August 18, 2009, http://tinyurl.com/lxbpes (accessed February 24, 2014).

3. Roxanne Nelson, "Soft Drink Consumption Linked to Pancreatic Cancer," Medscape.com, February 10, 2010, http://www.medscape.com/viewarticle/716806 (accessed February 11, 2014).

CHAPTER 12—THE PERFECT POMEGRANATE

1. María I. Gil et al., "Antioxidant Activity of Pomegranate Juice and Its Relationship With Phenolic Composition and Processing," *Journal of Agricultural and Food Chemistry* 48, no. 10 (2000): 4581–4589.

2. Salahuddin Ahmed et al., "*Punica granatum L.* Extract Inhibits IL-1ß-Induced Expression of Matrix Metalloproteinases by Inhibiting the Activation of MAP Kinases and NF-κB in Human Chondrocytes In Vitro," *Journal of Nutrition* 135 (2005): 2096–2102.

3. H. M. Kwak et al., "Beta-Secretase (BACE1) Inhibitors From Pomegranate Husk," *Archives Pharmacal Research* 28 (2005): 1328–1332.

4. MedlinePlus, "Pomegranate," http://tinyurl.com/7ox4rjp (accessed February 24, 2014).

5. M. Aviram et al., "Pomegranate Juice Consumption for Three Years by Patients With Carotid Artery Stenosis Reduces Common Carotid Intima-Media Thickness, Blood Pressure and LDL Oxidation," *American Journal of Clinical Nutrition* 23, no. 3 (June 2004): 423–433; Ahmad Esmaillzadeh et al., "Concentrated Pomegranate Juice Improves Lipid Profiles in Diabetic Patients With Hyperlipidemia," *Journal of Medicinal Food* 7, no. 3 (Fall 2004): 305–308; Marielle Kaplan et al., "Pomegranate Juice Supplementation to Atherosclerotic Mice Reduces Macrophage Lipid Peroxidation, Cellular Cholesterol Accumulation and Development of Atherosclerosis," *Journal of Nutrition* 131, no. 8 (August 1, 2001): 2082–2089.

6. Michael Aviram et al., "Pomegranate Juice Consumption Reduces Oxidative Stress, Atherogenic Modifications to LDL, and Platelet Aggregation: Studies in Humans and in Atherosclerotic Apolipoprotein E-Deficient Mice," *American Journal of Clinical Nutrition* 71, no. 5 (May 2000): 1062–1076.

7. Michael Aviram and Leslie Dornfeld, "Pomegranate Juice Consumption Inhibits Serum Angiotensin Converting Enzyme Activity and Reduces Systolic Blood Pressure," *Atherosclerosis* 158, no. 1 (September 2001):195–198.

8. T. D. Wilkins and A. S. Hackman, "Two Patterns of Neutral Steroid Conversion in the Feces of Normal North Americans," *Cancer Research* 34, no. 9 (1974): 2250–2254.

CHAPTER 13—OATMEAL: BREAKFAST OF CHAMPIONS

1. Eric R. Braverman, *Younger You* (New York: McGraw-Hill, 2006), 136.

2. Ibid., 137.

CHAPTER 14—PROTEIN POWER OF TURKEY

1. Information taken from *The Nutritive Value of Foods*, United States Department of Agriculture (USDA).

2. Harvard School of Public Health, "Protein: Moving Closer to Center Stage," http://tinyurl.com/nle2wzu (accessed February 24, 2014).

Chapter 15—The Strength of Salmon

1. G. M. Cole and S. A. Frautschy, "Docosahexaenoic Acid Protects From Amyloid and Dendritic Pathology in an Alzheimer's Disease Mouse Mode," *Nutrition Health* 18, no. 3 (2006): 249–259; P. Barberger-Gateau, C. Raffaitin, and L. Letenneur, "Dietary Patterns and Risk of Dementia: The Three-City Cohort Study," *Neurology* 69, no. 20 (2007): 1921–1930.
2. Penny M. Kris-Etherton, William S. Harris, and Lawrence J. Appel, "Fish Consumption, Fish Oil, Omega-3 Fatty Acids, and Cardiovascular Diseases," *Circulation* 106, no. 21 (November 19, 2002): 2747–2757; Erratum in *Circulation* 107, no. 3 (January 28, 2003): 512.
3. "Mercury Contamination in Fish," Natural Resources Defense Council, http://tinyurl.com/29wws3 (accessed February 24, 2014).
4. Gerard Judd, *Good Teeth From Birth to Death* (Glendale, AZ: EMR Labs, LLC, 2001).

Chapter 16—Citrus: Natural Sunshine

1. Béliveau and Gingras, *Foods to Fight Cancer*, 141.
2. Adam Hayashi, Aric C. Gillen, and James R. Lott, "Effects of Daily Oral Administration of Quercetin Chalcone and Modified Citrus Pectin on Implanted Colon-25 Tumor Growth in Balb-c Mice," *Alternative Medicine Review* 5, no. 6 (2000): 546–552.
3. As quoted in *Life Extension Magazine*, "A Report on Curcumin's Anti-cancer Effects," July 2002, http://eu.lef.org/en/magazines/77536 (accessed February 11, 2014).
4. Agency for Toxic Substances and Disease Registry, "Toxicological Profile for Chlordane," http://www.atsdr.cdc.gov/toxprofiles/tp.asp?id=355&tid=62 (accessed February 11, 2014).
5. Summarized on Medline Plus, "Migraine," U.S. National Library of Medicine and National Institutes of Health, http://www.nlm.nih.gov/medlineplus/migraine.html (accessed February 11, 2014). Information supplied by The National Institute of Neurological Disorders and Stroke.

6. University of Maryland Medical Center "Migraine Headache," http://tinyurl.com/73snx49 (accessed February 24, 2014).

CHAPTER 17—FAT-BURNING GREEN TEA

1. Bettuzzi S. School of Medicine, University of Parma, Italy; Jay Brooks, chairman, hematology/oncology, Ochsner Clinic Foundation Hospital, New Orleans; April 19, 2005, presentation, American Association for Cancer Research, annual meeting, Anaheim, CA.

2. Thomas A. Gasiewicz, "Receptor-Mediated Modulation of Gene Expression and Association With Biological and Toxic Responses," University of Rochester Medical School, August 20, 2009.

3. I. Takahashi et al., "Differences in the Influence of Tobacco Smoking on Lung Cancer Between Japan and the USA: Possible explanations for the 'Smoking Paradox' in Japan," *Public Health* 123, no. 6 (June 2009): 459–460.

4. S. Kuriyama et al., "Green Tea Consumption and Mortality Due to Cardiovascular Disease, Cancer, and All Causes in Japan: The Ohsaki Study," *Journal of the American Medical Association* 296, no. 10 (September 13, 2006): 1255–1265.

5. D. J. Maron et al., "Cholesterol-Lowering Effect of Theaflavin-Enriched Green Tea Extract: A Randomized Controlled Trial," *Archives of Internal Medicine* 163, no. 12 (June 23, 2003): 1448–1453.

CHAPTER 18—FLAX: TINY SEEDS, HUGE PAYOFF

1. S. E. McCann et al., "Dietary Lignan intakes and Risk of Pre- and Postmenopausal Breast Cancer," International Journal of Cancer 111, no. 3 (September 1, 2004): 440–443.

2. F. Boccardo et al., "Serum Enterolactone Levels and the Risk of Breast Cancer in Women with Palpable Cysts," European Journal of Cancer 40, no. 1 (January 2004): 84–89.

3. Milly Dawson, "Flaxseed: Protection Against Cancer, Heart Disease, and More," *Life Extension*, October 2008, http://tinyurl.com/odlgdlx (accessed February 24, 2014).

4. John R. Lee, Jesse Hanley, and Virginia Hopkins, *What Your Doctor May Not Tell You About Premenopause* (New York: Warner Books, 1999), 60.

Chapter 19—Dark Chocolate Dreams

1. Daniel J. DeNoon, "Dark Chocolate Is Healthy Chocolate," WebMD.com, August 27, 2003, http://tinyurl.com/3eyedb (accessed February 24, 2014).
2. Michelle Castillo, "Flavonol-Rich Dark Chocolate May Help Reduce Blood Pressure," CBS News, http://tinyurl.com/9h7k2wz (accessed February 24, 2014).
3. A. Buitrago-Lopez et al., "Chocolate Consumption and Cardiometabolic Disorders: Systematic Review and Meta-Analysis," *British Medical Journal* 343 (August 26, 2011).

Chapter 20—Yogurt: Your Gut Will Thank You

1. Phyllis A. Balch, *Prescription for Nutritional Healing*, third edition (New York: Avery, 2000), 74.

Chapter 21—Beans: Take a Bow

1. W. C. Willett et al., "Mediterranean Diet Pyramid: A Cultural Mode for Healthy Eating," *American Journal of Clinical Nutrition* 61, no. 6 (June 1995): 1402S–1406S.
2. Antonia Trichopoulou et al., "Cancer and the Mediterranean Dietary Traditions," *Cancer Epidemiology, Biomarkers & Prevention* 9 (September 2009): 869.
3. James W. Anderson, *Dr. Anderson's High-Fiber Fitness Plan* (Lexington, KY: University Press of Kentucky, 1994), 14.

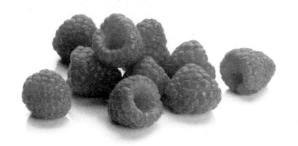
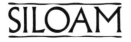

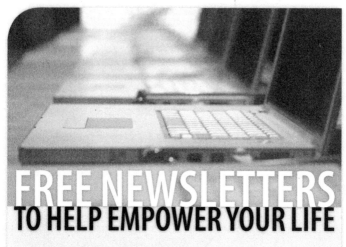

FREE NEWSLETTERS
TO HELP EMPOWER YOUR LIFE

Why subscribe today?

❏ **DELIVERED DIRECTLY TO YOU.** All you have to do is open your inbox and read.

❏ **EXCLUSIVE CONTENT.** We cover the news overlooked by the mainstream press.

❏ **STAY CURRENT.** Find the latest court rulings, revivals, and cultural trends.

❏ **UPDATE OTHERS.** Easy to forward to friends and family with the click of your mouse.

CHOOSE THE E-NEWSLETTER THAT INTERESTS YOU MOST:

- Christian news
- Daily devotionals
- Spiritual empowerment
- And much, much more

SIGN UP AT: **http://freenewsletters.charismamag.com**

8178